Social Capacity Building through Applied Theatre

T0384878

As experts in both applied theatre and education, Au Yi-Man and John O'Toole outline how applied theatre techniques can be used to support workers in the human services to develop crucial skills such as resilience, imagination, critical thinking, and reflection.

Highlighting under-emphasised skills and qualities in the human services professions, this book combines theory with context-specific practice to support capacity building across sectors. Drawing on a detailed study of NGO workers learning to use applied theatre techniques in professional development, the book offers insight into the learning and experiences of the participants and how these can be applied to future training programs. The book also provides a deeper understanding of how adult learners, from different backgrounds and levels of experience, approach their professional training. Rich with resources, the book features complete course examples, including theatre of the oppressed, process drama, and educational theatre, as core drama techniques.

Opening up new opportunities for applied theatre practitioners and educators, this book is a must-read for teachers in any human services field intending to use drama or applied theatre in their training.

Au Yi-Man is a practitioner, trainer, and researcher in applied theatre and drama education, the Executive Director of the Hong Kong Drama/Theatre and Education Forum (TEFO) and is on the editorial committee of *The Journal of Drama and Education in Asia* (DaTEAsia).

John O'Toole is an Honorary Professor and former Chair of Arts Education at the University of Melbourne, Australia and was lead author of the arts subject area of the Australian National Curriculum.

Learning Through Theatre: Dramatic Opportunities, Engagements and Challenges
Series Editors: John O'Toole and Kelly Freebody

This series commissions in-depth studies of the use of theatre and drama for the widest range of specific purposes – beyond entertainment itself – that involve learning. Contexts include formal educational settings such as schools and colleges, as well as social, communal, health, political, developing world, human services, war zones and commercial contexts. In the fields of applied theatre and drama education, three paradigms often define the purpose and the practice:

- drama as *art*
- drama as *education*
- drama as *social action and change*.

Books in the series tackle both the opportunities and the tensions among these paradigms: the developments, the challenges and the achievements in this still-growing field. Critical awareness and appraisal are a key feature, with some titles primarily grounded in theory and analysis, some more illustrative of good and bad practice. Authors include pioneers and established leaders as well as emerging practitioners and scholars.

Teaching and Learning Through Dramaturgy: Education as an Artful Engagement
Anna-Lena Østern

Applied Theatre in Paediatrics
Stories, Children and Synergies of Emotions
Persephone Sextou

Social Capacity Building through Applied Theatre
Developing Imagination, Emotional and Reflective Skills in the Human Services
Au Yi-Man and John O'Toole

For more information, please visit: https://www.routledge.com/Learning-Through-Theatre/book-series/LTT

Social Capacity Building through Applied Theatre

Developing Imagination, Emotional and Reflective Skills in the Human Services

Au Yi-Man and John O'Toole

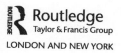
Routledge
Taylor & Francis Group

LONDON AND NEW YORK

Designed cover image: Guangzhou ShanDao Social Service Center

First published 2025
by Routledge
4 Park Square, Milton Park, Abingdon, Oxon OX14 4RN

and by Routledge
605 Third Avenue, New York, NY 10158

Routledge is an imprint of the Taylor & Francis Group, an informa business

© 2025 Au Yi-Man and John O'Toole

The right of Au Yi-Man and John O'Toole to be identified as authors of this work has been asserted in accordance with sections 77 and 78 of the Copyright, Designs and Patents Act 1988.

All rights reserved. No part of this book may be reprinted or reproduced or utilised in any form or by any electronic, mechanical, or other means, now known or hereafter invented, including photocopying and recording, or in any information storage or retrieval system, without permission in writing from the publishers.

Trademark notice: Product or corporate names may be trademarks or registered trademarks, and are used only for identification and explanation *without* intent to infringe.

British Library Cataloguing-in-Publication Data
A catalogue record for this book is available from the British Library

ISBN: 978-1-032-73045-5 (hbk)
ISBN: 978-1-032-73044-8 (pbk)
ISBN: 978-1-003-42638-7 (ebk)

DOI: 10.4324/9781003426387

Typeset in Times New Roman
by SPi Technologies India Pvt Ltd (Straive)

This book is dedicated
To the memory of our wise colleague, fellow-traveller,
and friend
CHRIS SINCLAIR
whose inspiration is found throughout these pages

Contents

Illustrations

Figure

Tables

Acknowledgements

The authors would like first and foremost to acknowledge the acumen, articulacy, confidence, and bravery of the Project participants in their responses to the applied theatre training workshop, and in giving permission for these to be shared publicly and openly in this book. We regret that it has not been possible to select and print all the responses of all the participants.

The authors would also like to thank the Graduate School of Education, the University of Melbourne, for the PhD scholarship and the resources the school provided. In addition, Yi-Man wishes to gratefully acknowledge the Institute for Civil Society, Sun Yat-Sen University, Guangzhou, for their kind offer to be the training workshop's supporting organisation.

Thanks to Tim Prentki for permission to modify and reprint a section from pp. 98–100 from O'Toole, J., Yi-Man, A., Baldwin, A., Cahill, H., & Chinyowa, K. (2015). Capacity building theatre (and vice versa). In Tim Prentki (Ed.). *Applied theatre: Development*. (pp. 98–100). Bloomsbury, in Chapter 10.

Yi-man's acknowledgments:

I would like to gratefully acknowledge my academic supervisors, Professor John O'Toole and Dr Christine Sinclair, and the thesis committee, Professor David Beckett, Associate Professor Kate Donelan and Professor Helen Cahill, for their continuous support, encouragement, patience, insightful comments and questions.

The origin of this project idea is indebted to Oxfam Hong Kong, which provided me with the opportunity to enter mainland China for the first time twenty years ago to give training in applied theatre. Since then, countless NGO participants have informed my learning about their work which contributed to my research. I would also like to express gratitude to Professor Chan K.M. for inspiring my interest in the development of NGOs in mainland China, which led me to dedicate a portion of my career to exploring NGO training projects in the country.

Initially, I thought that after completing my doctoral thesis, it would only be available for limited reading in the library. However, I was incredibly fortunate to receive the support of my mentor, Professor John O'Toole, who allowed my research to reach a wider audience. It was 'born' in Australia, submitted and selected as a Distinguished Dissertation by the American Alliance for Theatre Education in 2018, and later recommended by John for publication. I learned a lot during this rewriting process working alongside him. The appearance of this book not only allows the research findings to continue engaging in dialogue with professionals worldwide but also serves as a precious gift exchanged between John and me. I am truly indescribably grateful to John, my dear teacher, mentor, senior colleague, and lifelong friend, for his immeasurable support and trust.

Preface

Preamble

We should start by explaining just what we mean by 'applied theatre' and 'human services' as each of these umbrella terms may be familiar to only one portion of our readership. Applied theatre is a phrase coined in the early 1990s, and now widely accepted, to define the growing movement of people using theatre and drama practices for purposes beyond entertainment, not in conventional theatres or drama studios, but in locations and settings that relate to those purposes. Many of those purposes are found within in our other umbrella term: the services and professions that exist to fulfil human, social needs in communities of all kinds.

In many of these fields, education and learning in their broadest sense often replace the entertainment that is the primary purpose of conventional drama and theatre, along with caring and health, community building or restoring, and any context dependent on human relations. Applied theatre has already found its purposes right across this vast field of human social endeavour, which is why it is still growing fast across the globe, and gradually becoming recognised more widely. Below, and in Chapter 3, we shall explain this more fully.

The essential soft skills

Imagination, and *emotional intelligence*, and *reflective skills*, the keywords of our subtitle, are qualities that are more and more essential for human services workers in our contemporary world, from nurses and teachers to health workers and carers, and from war zones to human resources (HR) departments. However, it is quite rare for them to form a major part of the appointment criteria, or the service workers' training. In fact, they are terms unused or unvalued in some of those service professions and also some parts of the globe, and invariably subordinate to certificated cognitive knowledge and skills. To them we might add *empathic skills*, *resilience*, *critical thinking*, *resourcefulness*, and *the ability to listen* – with the eyes as well as the ears. However, throughout the fields of human services, all these words provide demands and challenges that many workers struggle to meet or measure up to within their fields. Human services, by definition, are full of the problems, the challenges and the unpredictability of humans in social and community situations. These soft skills are all prime characteristics of applied theatre, core elements of our craft. We will demonstrate through theory, derived directly from the evidence of our lead author's practice, that they are exactly what can make drama, and especially applied theatre, a crucial and sustainable addition to the basic training of workers right across the human services.

As every thinking actor, dramatist, director, and stage manager, ancient and modern, has always known, *empathy* and *imagination; dialogue* and *listening; discipline and sensitivity; resilience* and *resourcefulness, quick and critical thinking* and *reflective capacity* are all vital components of theatrecraft.

- The basic dramatic act is to put oneself into another's shoes in an *imagined* world – to identify and *empathise* with the wearer of those shoes, understand them *emotionally* as well as cognitively, and maybe also to distance oneself and *reflect* on that character and their world.
- Drama is a group and an ensemble art. Its basic mode of expression is *dialogue*, action and interaction creating a social situation to bring that imagined world to life for its audience.
- Every piece of drama or theatre (whether for an external audience or just the participants) is therefore also the artistry of ensemble, where each player must *listen to each other*, play their part in the whole, and exactly that. Training *sensitivity* to the whole group and all its members is part of this, and that is what rehearsals are for.
- This is the first place where *discipline* comes in. That's just half of it. Apart from the obvious disciplines of learning one's role and one's lines – if scripted – and knowing where to be and when, theatre discipline is quite as crucially the ability to listen and respond. To the ensemble and director, of course, but the ensemble is not the whole, or even necessarily the most important part of the dramatic experience. Even if separated by a 'fourth wall' and the one-way performance conventions of a traditional theatre genre, there are the consumers (a word now frequently used in human services for what used to be called clients or patients, and in theatre is still called audience). They come with expectations and their own context of experience. Good actors and ensembles will reach out through that wall to check on the audience's reactions and fine-tune their performance accordingly. In applied theatre, that quality becomes central, because, unlike for a traditional performance, the audience is not there just for a good time; they have a specific purpose in being there, and the ensemble of theatre makers is gathered to fulfil that purpose. Some audiences may not even be there voluntarily, such as children captive in an in-school theatre-in-education (TiE) program, or villagers lured or driven to the performance space for a lesson on sanitation or HiV-AIDS.
- And this is exactly why *resilience* and *critical thinking* are so important, much more so to the applied theatre worker than the conventional actor,

who will be constrained by their contract to complete the performance no matter what effect their sensitive tweaking has, and only be faced afterwards with the negative comments of onlookers or reviewers. Those kinds of comments have given rise to the cliché in the professional theatre that an actor needs 'the soul of a fairy and the hide of a rhino'. This truism becomes an inescapable and immediate truth for applied theatre performers when their audience just gets up and walks out, or throws objects and abuse, and the sponsors as a result cancel the whole program.

- Any applied theatre worker worth their salt does not waste time on blame or recrimination, but accepts the audience's verdict, even gratefully, and goes into *critical thinking*, analysing why the program's intentions did not match the expectations or comfort level of the audience and give them a good time. This will be accompanied by *reflection* on themselves, *and replanning* of an improved program.

Human services workers, like applied theatre workers, mostly do not choose their consumers, and have to deal with the expectations and tolerance levels they are faced with, and the same kinds of missteps. A human services worker must be constantly learning, and often ensuring their consumers are learning too. At its most basic, too, all drama involves some kind of shared learning – a new story or a new take on an old one; or new insights into human behaviour; often even messages and questions deliberately crafted into the dramatic experience for the audience. Over the last half-century, drama educators have been developing those raw natural qualities of the art form into a way of learning, a pedagogy initially designed for schools and adopted by applied theatre for wider community use. This pedagogy radically disrupts the central traditional premise of both orthodox schooling and theatre itself, that the act of schooling, like a conventional play, is an essentially one-way performance delivered by people who know to audiences of those who don't.

Schooling systems and theatres are still struggling to free themselves from that trap. For more than a century, John Dewey and all the following generations of constructivist educators – Vygotsky, Bruner, Eisner et al. (add your own favourite progressive educator) – and thousands and thousands of projects and books, have demonstrated conclusively that the central figure in education is not the teacher(s) but the learner(s). The teachers – and their accoutrements – do not perform to the children; instead, they engage in a two-way performance of shared learning. This is dialogic, and basically democratic, sharing of power.

Theatre too, over approximately the same time period, and primarily driven by the study of children's play and the possibilities of audience interaction, has discovered that the central figure in theatre is not necessarily the artist but the audience. Dramatic experience and performance can equally be two-way, dialogic and democratic. In Chapter 3, we shall explore the derivation of these discoveries in both fields, but together, they form the basis for contemporary applied theatre and much drama education. Applied theatre now applies itself to almost any community of need, just as the human services industries do. This is often through non-government organisations (NGOs), quasi- – or partially – officially funded organisations (QUANGOs), and voluntary providers the world over. For most of them, no professional training may be available, let alone one that develops capacity in the 'soft skills' that are the subject of this book.

Researching soft skills

Finding methods of developing capacity in these soft skills, and then identifying whether, why, and how much the methods are effective is, of course, much harder than measuring development and learning in cognitive knowledge and skills, which is why they are still often overlooked, undervalued, or dismissed as 'unknowable' in professional training programs right across the human services. However, this does not mean they are unknowable. They are often instantly recognisable in the effect they have on the people and contexts involved. In theatre as in human services contexts, live experience says what figures and books cannot. Everybody knows instinctively when they are inspired, challenged, or comforted, or the penny drops for them. The proof of the pudding is in the eating. The evidence of the senses can provide the proof of the pudding, either immediately in the taste and smell, or later in feeling its ability to sustain. Beyond the literal wisdom of this old metaphor, the most valuable senses for **our** research are the eyes and ears, and this book is all about seeing and listening to live experience, and then reflecting on it.

Knowing this both instinctively and cognitively, and from her own experience, our lead author, Au Yi-Man, gathered a remarkable group of applied theatre workshop participants from across a range of human services contexts. In two ways they were remarkable: first, they were all trainers themselves, so they could see the whole process from the dual position of deliverer and consumer; second, because what they had in common was working for NGOs, so they came from a diverse range of human services settings. She crafted for them, and shared in, a rich, complex, and challenging experience of applied theatre. Throughout, she trusted the evidence of her eyes and ears, and her own ability to reflect on and interpret the experience. For this reason, we have not deleted the participants' own words from Yi-Man's original study, as would be more usual for a book, but, on the contrary, highlighted the wisest and most revealing of them so that they form a fascinating grass-roots basis for our guidelines. From the author and the participants in dialogue together, a proto-dramatic narrative emerges, where those participants become the reader's familiar friends. They provide a mosaic of impressive stories of personal development, revealing the importance of imaginative, emotional, and reflective growth, to complement the participants' growing cognitive understanding and experience. We hope you will be as inspired by these stories as we have been, that we will then use to transform into general principles and guidelines for your, and others', practice.

Abbreviations

DE/DiE	Drama education/drama-in-education
HiV-AIDS	Virus causing acquired autoimmune deficiency syndrome (AIDS)
HR	Human Relations (Department)
IDEA	International Drama/Theatre and Education Association
INTRAC	An international organisation to promote civil society building
NGO	Non-government organisation
NPO	Non-profit organisation
Oxfam	International organisation for famine and poverty relief
Quango	Quasi-autonomous non-government organisation
TtT	Train-the-trainer programs
TiE	Theatre-in-education
TfD	Theatre for development
TO	Theatre of the oppressed
UN, UNO	United Nations Organisation

Part I
The background

1   Starting my quest in China

My credentials for the journey

I knew nothing about Chinese non-government organisations (NGOs) until my first job in mainland China. As an experienced applied theatre practitioner from Hong Kong, in 2004 I was invited to co-facilitate a one-day applied theatre workshop in Beijing with a group of NGO workers from different provinces organised by the Hong Kong chapter of the international charity Oxfam. At that time, Oxfam had set up a new team in China to promote Development Education throughout NGOs. In the Oxfam workshop, participants in small groups created dramas on development issues. We chose one out of them to demonstrate a Forum Theatre process, which will be defined and explained in detail later. The workshop received much positive feedback from participants as well as the organiser. We found that there are many compatible elements between development education and applied theatre. Both value the qualities of participation, interaction, experiential learning, expression, dialogue and action.

Oxfam became at that time an important supporter of the promotion of applied theatre in China. Over the next five years, there were six Train-the-Trainer (TtT) workshops on applied theatre, in five of which I was involved. Another seven projects organised by NGO partners included applied theatre techniques as part of the training. Three People's Theatre Forums were funded. In 2007, Oxfam supported 30 NGO workers from China to attend the International Drama/Theatre and Education Association (IDEA) World Congress held in Hong Kong. It is not entirely clear why Oxfam decided to run such courses for NGO workers at this time, but the known high burnout rates of NGO workers, and their lack of specific training for their functions in their NGOs, were among the factors in Oxfam's recognition that NGO leaders and trainers needed some additional training.

Apart from the collaboration with Oxfam, I was regularly invited by other local or international organisations to work with Chinese NGO workers in workshops lasting from one to four days. Usually I found myself working for nationwide training programs for all NGOs, but sometimes I worked for an individual NGO as part of its professional development. In the following six

DOI: 10.4324/9781003426387-2

years, I conducted around 18 TtT workshops in China and worked with nearly 450 NGO workers from a range of NGOs. Some participants stayed in touch with me, actively applying theatre in their work. They were keen on further learning and looking for whatever opportunities they could find to gain more understanding. With most, I lost contact; I have no idea whether they continued to use applied theatre in their work, and, if so, how effective it was. All of this first-hand contact was beginning to give me glimpses of insight into NGOs, and the challenges the workers faced.

For those next few years, the connection between development and applied theatre in China thrived. Applied theatre training continued to be organised in the NGO field, with the techniques not only integrated into the work on development education, but applied in different aspects of the field. Several applied theatre practitioners were invited from overseas to provide training for the local communities. Some NGOs even started to train their clients or consumers to use applied theatre.

Questions raised on my journey

All of this raised further questions for me. Unlike other places in Asia such as Taiwan, Hong Kong and Japan, where the participants and trainers in applied theatre come mainly from teaching or formal social work domains, in mainland China NGO workers, with some social workers, were the most numerous participants, because of the funding sources. They were obviously keen to learn any new skills for their work. They treated the training as a capacity-building opportunity, which is where this phrase started to resonate more and more for me. As one of the earliest applied theatre practitioners working in China, I began to wonder: does applied theatre training contribute to capacity building for NGO workers? If so, how, and what factors might support or inhibit its effective application?

While there was rarely any question of the personal commitment of the participants, I began to see some of the challenges they faced. These were challenges in their daily practice, and legacies, assumptions and deficits in their training – and their whole educational background. I became aware of some serious problems endemic to the field of NGO services throughout China and the personnel within them. Government statistics, which I started to explore, indicated for instance that the very high burn-out rate of NGO workers and organisers was leading to a more shifting population than desirable. This might have been partly too because of their low incomes, and the lack of career prospects for young people.

By 2009 I had decided to really explore this field in proper depth, and also to use my applied theatre experience, not in more ad hoc workshops, but in a systematic investigation into the impact and sustainability of applied theatre for a range of NGOs and their workers. This would include practical fieldwork as well as a thorough analysis of the beliefs, values and practices of contemporary NGOs in a range of fields.

NGOs in China

Non-government organisation (NGO) is a term coined and developed in the West. It first appeared in a United Nations document in 1945. Because of the different natures, boundaries and orientations of the organisations it encompasses, it lacks a unified definition. However, NGOs 'generally share the common properties of being non-governmental, non-commercial, public and voluntary' (Wang & Liu, 2009: 6).

The concept started to become used in China in the mid-1980s. Although the term NGO itself was used from the earliest times, many other terms were used in the field dependent on the legal status and the emphasis of the organisations. K.M. Chan (2005: 24) mentioned that legally established NGOs existed in China in the form of 'registered intermediate organisations'. However, at the time of my project, there were three types of registered groups, respectively called 'social organisations' (*shehui tuanti*), 'non-governmental non-profit units' (*minban feiqiye danwei*), and 'foundations' (*jijin hui*). Many people called unregistered NGOs 'grassroots NGOs' to highlight their bottom-up nature. NPO (non-profit organisations) and groups of volunteers were other popular terms. A little later, the term 'philanthropic organisation' gained currency, partly in order to increase the organisation's acceptability to public and entrepreneurial sponsors.

This multiple nomenclature draws attention to the confusing and sensitive identities of NGOs in China. Although there were (and still are) different names employed for different purposes, in this book I will employ NGO as a general term to refer to any of the organisations and fields the participants in my research experiment were working in.

We need to delve a little more into the history to understand the background and significant scale of NGO development. As everyone knows, starting from the late 1970s, China dramatically changed its economic structure by expanding the scope of markets and private ownership, which in turn set in motion a vast process of social transformation. This created a new landscape of wealth distribution, which widened the gap between the rich and the poor. As a by-product, the rapid economic growth entailed numerous layoffs, the down-sizing of government bureaucracy and the shedding of many government functions. Fifty years later, this changed status quo is inescapable. The functions of traditional work units became eroded. Those economic reforms brought even more social problems, like unemployment, inequality, and increased pollution. At the same time they greatly reduced the state's commitment to welfare. This then generated the need to expand the social organisation sector to take on these functions on behalf of society. On the other hand, the general improvement in living standards, and the increased time and space allowed for private and social lives, became another driving force that created opportunities – and the necessity – for NGOs to develop.

From the 1990s, the Chinese government decided that 'small government, big society' would be a trend in its political reform. Social organisations would be encouraged to play a more active role in society. NGOs started to attract broad attention (Wang & Liu, 2009). Different areas of the economy opening up favoured the development of a burgeoning NGO sector. In the last three decades, according to the official website of the Ministry of Civil Affairs (www. mca.gov.cn), the number of registered NGOs expanded significantly from 107,304 in 1991 to 891,206 in 2022. (This is the number of organisations themselves, remember, not individual workers.)

However, the Chinese government did not really allow NGOs to expand freely. Instead, it imposed strict legal and administrative controls over them. The 1998 regulation had stipulated that only one organisation of its kind was allowed to register within the same administrative region. This largely limited the growth of social organisations in China, including NGOs. The high bar registration system made it difficult for a large number of NGOs to gain legal status and so they remained unregistered, where they could only be a subsidiary to the registered social organisations. Although the government relaxed the legal and administrative controls on some of the service-oriented NGOs, the advocacy groups and NGOs working in sensitive areas such as labour or human rights issues were still under close scrutiny and some of them suppressed. In 2016 another new law made it harder for overseas organisations either to register or provide support to local organisations ever since.

(NB. This was the NGO landscape at the time of my project, but for the history, it should be noted that this landscape has changed further. In the last ten years, the Chinese Government has extensively increased its national control in every area. Government is not 'small' anymore. And it supports more government-funded and registered social workers organisations to provide social services instead of independent NGOs.)

Apart from the difficulty with registration, the lack of funding and resources of all kinds were another two major predicaments facing the development of NGOs. The government subsidy only went to the registered NGOs or their subsidiaries. As the government was withdrawing its financial commitment to social organisations, registered NGOs turned to outside sources. Before 2019's compulsory registration, the financial situation was even worse for the unregistered and grassroots NGOs, due to a lack of bargaining power to compete with registered or bigger NGOs. Chan (2005) also notes the serious difficulties for NGOs in raising donations from communities that lacked either trust in them or public-spiritedness, while the state did not provide tax deductions or other institutional support that would encourage donations. Although the scene was changing, with new laws in 2004 and 2016 which allowed the set-up of private foundations to increase local funding sources for NGOs, their resources were still limited. Furthermore the above-mentioned 2016 Overseas NGO Law forced numerous international NGOs to leave China, which further cut off financial support to local organisations. The unstable financial sources made Chinese NGOs put most of their efforts into striving to survive.

Lack of capacity, on the part of both the organisations themselves, and also of their staff, has been another major constraint on the development of

Chinese NGOs. There was widespread criticism of NGOs' deficiencies in resource mobilisation, organisation and management skills, coordination and crisis response capacity. NGOs being a relatively new profession in China, there were no prior reference points about how to run a social organisation. According to Wang and Liu (2009), investigations showed that in NGO societies and foundations, more than 90% of employees had received no professional training. In more recent years, it seems there has been greater concern about NGO training, but it is still far from enough. Furthermore, the general wage level was too low to attract talented professionals entering the field. Naturally, this both hindered NGOs from providing quality service to the public and made it difficult to gain credibility for their healthy development.

NGO capacity building in China

According to one of the leading Chinese NGO scholars, Professor Zhu Jiang-Gang (personal communication, 2011), starting from the late 1990s there were three stages of development of capacity building in China. The first was the directly imported stage. The training just simply duplicated the courses from Western NGOs. The second was the critical and reflective stage. NGOs found that the 'imported methods' were not fully fit and appropriate for local practices and started to search for their own ways of capacity building. The third was the adaptation and creation stage. Local NGOs tried to localise the Western training courses as well as to create new courses. By 2011, there were generally two channels of training: first, an increasing number of government-accredited degree courses provided by universities; second, non-accredited courses and workshops provided by local and/or international NGOs. Because of the high prerequisites and the cost, only an elite few could get training via the first channel. For most NGOs, the second channel was their main source of training opportunities. The first local NGO training organisation was founded in 1998 in Beijing. Since then, an increasing number of foundations expanded their support for capacity building organisations and programs, until about 8–9 NGO support organisations had been set up in different cities to provide training (Zhu 2011).

In general, the training content was focused on the organisational level. A 2011 textbook on capacity building, published by the National Management of Social Organisations Bureau – which since 2016 has just been called the Social Organisation Bureau (Shèhuì zǔzhī guǎnlǐ jú) – identified the capacities of social organisations to include the abilities for internal governance, strategic management, fundraising, financial management, human resources management (including staff and volunteer management), social marketing and public relations, project management and creditability management. When I reviewed the course contents of different NGO support organisations, their programs did appear to cover a large proportion of these management-driven capacity-building aims. For training at an individual level, some organisations offered training courses in facilitation skills and leadership training to organisational heads, though not their staff. Although there were a few programs in recent years that have tried to provide relatively longer training to individuals, at the time of my conducting my fieldwork in China the courses were still predominantly short-term, from a few hours to a week's duration. These one-off courses usually had no follow-up or continuous relationship between the trainers and trainees afterwards.

When I considered these practices in China, it seemed that the course designs always reflected the rationales of the training providers, rather than the customers. Reviewing the subjects of the courses provided by most training organisations, it was clear that their first priority was to help NGOs to survive. They believed good management and accountability are the keys to sustain the organisation and get support from foundations and the public. That was why their training programs tended to focus on the organisational level. Some had broader aims, concerned to strengthen particular beliefs and values of NGOs in order to build a stable civil society in China. Their training content included considerable exploration of the development of the NGO and its function in society. Apart from those priorities, the training might be directed by the funders' agendas. For example, the first applied theatre workshop I conducted in China was instituted by Oxfam to introduce participatory strategies for promoting development education.

Since the cost of staff training was usually not covered by funding, a lack of resources made it very difficult for any individual NGO to design and create their own training program. In 2009, I interviewed 30 NGOs in five cities across the country. The organisations' heads normally had no concrete plan for internal training. For them, 'training' meant informal mentoring and learning by doing. Staff very seldom received well-planned and systematic group training and sometimes not even immediate support. So, they had to rely for their professional growth mainly on independent learning on the job. I understood that the urge to survive among NGOs and the urge to strengthen civil society were core concerns in this developmental stage. However, I did wonder to what extent the dominant courses on teaching about how to run an efficient social organisation could really help to nurture a person working in the field. So, how is an individual NGO worker to maintain good practice, when they are working in such an unstable internal and external (political and social) situation that lacks training and support?

Although there were extensive reports on Chinese NGOs starting from the mid-1990s, the literature, including the most up-to-date contributions, reflected efforts to understand NGOs from the perspective of political science or sociology. These studies always focused on a state or organisational level, for example, exploring state–society relations and Chinese modern organisations, exploring the relationship between civil participation and NGO development, and exploring the development of the NGO and its potential influence for democratisation in China.

A number of scholars did mention 'capacity building' as one of the major difficulties for the Chinese NGOs, because the impact of capacity building was still poorly documented, and there was no clear and agreed definition of what capacities needed building, and for whom. Capacity building is an imported concept in China, not fully understood nor widely implemented. Though Chinese NGOs were seeking ways for improving localised practice, they did recognise the importance of capacity building. Because of the relative absence of discussion of the topic at the time, I decided it would be useful in my project - and now for the reader - to explore the concept of capacity building from Western literature and its implications.

Notions of capacity building

The language of 'capacity building' has become ubiquitous among international funding agencies in the twenty-first century, referring to both government and non-governmental organisations (Hartwig et al., 2008). In the NGO literature, the word gained a 'buzzword' status. However, capacity building remained a concept of enormous generality and vagueness. It was a catch-all concept and there was already widespread concern that in encompassing everything it lacked coherence. It can be a process, an outcome, a strategy, a methodology, an approach or an activity. The various definitions of 'capacity' at the time range from a description of an external intervention to a discussion of a process of change: from macro to micro level of support, including 'soft' (motivational and processual) and/or 'hard' (technical) elements.

Capacities for beneficiaries

Generally, there were – and still are – two areas of discussion on capacity building in the literature. The first is about capacity building for the beneficiaries. According to Joe Bolger (2000), over the past fifty years with the dominant role of donor-led projects, inadequate attention to long-term 'capacity' issues has resulted in limited sustainable impact in priority areas. Leanne Black (2003) criticises the dominant discourse for concentrating mainly on technical and communications interests. This reflects the imperatives of traditional social systems theory, which identified with 'functionalist' constructs of capacity-building discourse that cannot help to reduce poverty. He points out how poorly represented are emancipatory interests which Habermas describes as 'the human need for freedom from subjection, oppression and alienation, and this feeds politically liberating activities' (Moore cited in Black, 2003). Increasingly, there is a call for a shift in the conceptualisation of 'capacity building' from a mechanistic resource-transfer mentality to a systemic understanding of, and approach to, change. So, as Deborah Eade stresses, '*capacity building is an approach to development*, not something separate from it. It is a response to the multi-dimensional processes of change, not a set of discrete or pre-packaged technical interventions intended to bring about a pre-defined outcome' (1997; original italics). Whatever approaches people choose to build capacity, there is consensus

that any capacity-building initiative should be: owned and driven by participants; organised yet flexible; long-term and process-oriented; based on
shared values and building on strengths; context-specific; enhanced by strong
working relationships; and multi-faceted. One of the typical views on development in the field:

> Development is about women and men becoming empowered to bring
> about positive changes in their lives; about personal growth together with
> public action; about both the process and the outcome of challenging
> poverty, oppression, and discrimination; and about the realization of
> human potential through social and economic justice. Above all, it is
> about the process of transforming lives, and transforming societies.
>
> (Eade, 1997: 24)

The classic saying in the field, 'Give a man a fish, feed him for a day; teach him
how to fish, feed him for a lifetime', is why development practitioners have shifted
to a more long-lasting, process-oriented and participative way of capacity
building.

Capacities for each NGO

The second capacity-building discussion in the literature is about the NGOs
themselves. According to Rick James (2002), capacity building within NGOs
can occur on four different levels: individual, organisational, inter-
organisational, and societal. Different levels of intervention can focus on different goals, from capacity building as an end in itself to as a means to broader
ends. Capacity building will be seen as an end in itself if its initiatives focus
just on the provision of material and/or technical support which enable NGOs
to carry out their immediate goals of project-related services. At the other end
of the spectrum are those initiatives which treat NGOs purely as a means to
achieving broader ends to create a strong and vibrant democratic culture
(Hudock, 1999: 33–34). These levels are in fact inter-linked. You cannot build
a more vibrant civil society without developing an effective coalition of
organisations. A good inter-organisational relationship relies on different single and strong organisations. This leads 'organisational development' to
become a popular subject in NGO capacity-building interventions. However,
organisations consist of people and organisational change is based on individual change – as James (2002: 6) points out. INTRAC, a leading international NPO, makes the analogy that capacity-building intervention is like a
drop of rain that lands in water, creating the ripples that flow outward to
bring about change on a broader level. NGO workers whose capacities are
enhanced at personal level will have potential power to act on and affect their
environment and, ultimately, may trigger social change. The importance of
the individual level of capacity building is also a key for providing better service to the beneficiaries.

What about capacities for real people?

From the above, the reader can see, as I was beginning to see, that there was a clearly growing concern with the concept of people-centred development in capacity building both with beneficiaries and within the NGOs. Inclusive language, like cooperation, participation, ownership, empowerment, multi-stakeholder dialogue, power-sharing and democratic processes permeates the capacity-building discourse. I came to believe that the relationship between capacity building for the beneficiaries and capacity building for NGOs is inseparable. So, I started to ask myself as I approached my project, how can these concepts be put into practice? Can NGO workers build capacities in others that they don't have themselves? How can they equip themselves with the capacity-building skills for participatory people-centred development? As change agents working in 'a risky, murky, messy business, with unpredictable and unquantifiable outcomes, uncertain methodologies, contested objectives, many unintended consequences, little credit to its champions and long time-lags' (Peter Morgan, cited in Lusthaus et al., 1999), the total capacity required of them is inevitably a big challenge. The personal nature of change is complex but necessary.

> [The human dimension of] capacity building requires shifts in people's behaviours and attitudes…Capacity building is as much about letting go of the old as it is about taking on the new. Change, and therefore capacity building, is not an easy thing for anyone. It engages people's emotions, their fears and desires…Capacity building also alters people's relationships with others and thereby touches on very sensitive issues of power.
>
> (James, 2002: 3)

Critical and analytical thinking is essential to any transformative process. It needs to be allied to something more fundamental and intuitive, some form of sensitivity, inquisitiveness, creativity, or change in consciousness. Peter Morgan (2006: 8–16) identifies the following five core capabilities:

- **the capability to act and self-organise**: to do that with attitudes and self-perceptions which come from a complex blend of motivation, commitment, space, confidence, security, meaning, and values and identity;
- **the capability to generate development results**: a. to improve their own capabilities and to help develop the capabilities of those with whom they work, and b. to fulfil programmatic goals;
- **the capability to relate**: to work with other actors within the contexts and to form alliances or/and partnerships;
- **the capability to adapt and self-renew**: to master the change and the adoption of new ideas;
- **the capability to achieve coherence**: to integrate structures inside the system.

All these are abilities, as we see from the preface, are equally essential for applied theatre workers in community settings.

Allan Kaplan (2000: 524–525) goes on helpfully and imaginatively to identify new abilities to develop people's thinking, rather than skills, to build capacity:

- the ability to find the right question which may enable an organisation to take the next step on its path of development, and to hold a question so that it functions as a stimulus to exploration rather than demanding an immediate solution;
- the ability to hold the tension generated by ambiguity and uncertainty rather than seek immediate resolution;
- the ability to observe accurately and objectively, to listen deeply, so that invisible realities of the organisation become manifest;
- the ability to use metaphor and imagination to overcome resistance to change, to enable an organisation to see itself afresh, and to stimulate creativity;
- the ability to help others to overcome cynicism and despair and to kindle enthusiasm;
- integrity, and the ability to generate the trust which alone will allow the organisation and its members to really 'speak' and reveal themselves;
- the ability to reflect honestly on one's own interventions, and to enable others to do the same;
- the ability to 'feel' into the 'essence' of a situation;
- the ability to empathise (not sympathise) so that both compassion and confrontation can be used with integrity in helping an organisation to become unstuck;
- the ability to conceptualise, and thus to analyse strategy with intelligence.

My voyage of discovery (research)

Kaplan elegantly suggests that people working in the NGO field are:

'artists of the invisible', continually having to deal with ambiguity and paradox, uncertainty in the turbulence of change, new and unique situations coming to us from out of a future of which we have had as yet little experience. This more radical response would imply that we need to develop a resourcefulness out of which we can respond, rather than being trained in past solutions, in fixed mindsets, and trained behaviours which replicate particular patterns and understandings instead of freeing us to respond uniquely to unique situations.

(Kaplan 2000: 524)

The idea that capacity building is an art, not a science, captured me. And, as an art it is likely to be a complex voyage of personal and collective discovery that evolves over time. This was all I needed to clinch my determination to see whether my own art of applied theatre could have any impact, however small, on the mighty gaps in NGO understanding and practice we have been exploring above, and provide any guide to capacity building in those qualities described in the subtitle of the book.

To meet the demand for increased capacities in people-centred development, the organisational level can only make an inadequate response, because, as I said earlier, an organisation consists of individual workers. It is hard for an organisation to have all these democratic and participative values without having their staff equipped with the abilities to learn, to reflect, to engage, to feel and to imagine, etc. These discrepancies were particularly part of the Chinese NGOs scene, which paid little attention to any discussion about individual workers' capacity building. In my experience as an applied theatre practitioner, coming into China to conduct training workshops with NGO workers, it had become apparent that applied theatre shares many similar values with a people-centred approach to NGO capacity building. Applied theatre has established practices in which exploring the potential for human change is possible through structuring a dialogic, open, aesthetic, interactive, and reflective space to create multiple embodied experiences for participants. They have been central to our literature even from before the term applied theatre was coined. Later writers have added substance, structure, and nuance to those powerful statements of principle, as we shall demonstrate in Chapter 3.

Therefore, my belief that there should be a place for applied theatre to contribute to NGO capacity building was my prime reason for starting the study, and led to the formulation of my research question, which was focused in my particular context, though this book will show that it has implications far beyond China, and beyond NGOs.

Does applied theatre training contribute to capacity building for NGO workers in China? If so, how, and what factors might support or inhibit its effective application?

In 2009, the University of Melbourne gave me a PhD scholarship to pursue this question, which completely occupied me for more than half the next decade. My study adopted a blend of action research and reflective practitioner research as its methodology, which, just like applied theatre, are both participatory processes bringing together action and reflection, theory and practice, in participation with others.

The project was based on fieldwork consisting of an applied theatre training workshop with a group of Chinese NGO workers. Through a careful and systematic inquiry guided by action research, I wanted to investigate how the design and implementation of an applied theatre training workshop might impact on NGO workers' learning and sustained capacity building. The training workshop lasted for three months, divided into three phases, where one selected genre of applied theatre, *theatre of the oppressed* (TO), *process drama* and *participatory theatre* – all to be explained – was introduced in each phase. The iterative process of doing action research generated plenty of diverse data from phase to phase of the action-based cycles, that informed both the immediate teaching and also my post-project analysis.

In addition, as a facilitator I was myself a participant insider in the training process, one whose thoughts and actions strongly influenced the participants' learning. This provided me unexpectedly with some of the most definitive insights of the project, not just for developing my own practice, but in re-evaluating the critical importance of the project's facilitator, and the necessary qualities which that person or those persons must have. In order to gain more understanding of my own practice as an applied theatre training facilitator, in this study I also implemented reflective practice to document my thoughts underpinning the practice and the depth of my own reflection about the teaching method. These were methods that not only prompted continuous self-inquiry but much more importantly also opened a dialogic, creative, and human space for the investigation of NGO and other human services workers' capacities and skills within an applied theatre practice. Furthermore, through this research, I wanted to find out the necessary considerations for planning training workshops as well as mapping my impact on others' learning.

That became the basis of this book: my broader intention to make explicit for others too the process of learning about and through applied theatre, in order to contribute both to the practice of capacity building – especially for individual human services workers – and to show that applied theatre training can provide trainees with an effective pedagogy for human change.

References

Black, L. (2003). Critical review of the capacity building literature and discourse. *Development in Practice, 13*(1), 116–120.

Bolger, J. (2000). Capacity development: Why, what and how. *Capacity Development Occasional Series, 1*(1). Retrieved from http://nsagm.weebly.com/uploads/1/2/0/3/12030125/capacity_development_cida.pdf

Chan, K. M. (2005). The development of NGOs a post-totalitarian regime: The case of China. In P. R. Weller (Ed.), *Civil life, globalization, and political change in Asia: organizing between family and state* (pp. 20–41). London: Routledge.

Eade, D. (1997). *Capacity-building: An approach to people-centred development.* Oxfam, UK and Ireland.

Hartwig, K. A., Humphries, D., & Matebeni, Z. (2008). Building capacity for AIDS NGOs in southern Africa: Evaluation of a pilot initiative. *Health Promotion International, 23*(3), 251–259.

Hudock, A. C. (1999). *NGOs and civic society: democracy by proxy?* Malden, UK: Blackwell.

James, R. (2002). *People and change: Exploring capacity building in NGOs.* INTRAC Publications, Great Britain.

Kaplan, A. (2000). Capacity building: Shifting the paradigms of practice. *Development in Practice, 10*(3 & 4), 517–525.

Lusthaus, C., Adrien, M.-H., & Perstinger, M. (1999). Capacity development: Definitions, issues and implications for planning, monitoring and evaluation. *Universalia Occasional Paper, 35*. Retrieved from https://www.universalia.com/files/occas35.pdf

Morgan, P. (2006). *The concept of capacity (Draft version).* European Centre for Development Policy Management. Retrieved from http://ecdpm.org/wp-content/uploads/2006-The-Concept-of-Capacity.pdf

Wang, M., & Liu, Q. (2009). Analyzing China's NGO Development System. *The China Nonprofit Review, 1*(1), 5–35.

Zhu, J.-G. (2011). *Chinese NGOs.* Personal communication with the author.

2 Teaching adults

Preamble

In the previous chapter, Yi-Man mentioned that there are different kinds and levels of capacity building which are relevant to NGO training. Although her applied theatre training workshops were in the first instance an approach for individual NGO workers, we were both aware that the broader aspects which had to be considered for their effective capacity building were equally applicable in a wide range of training and adult education purposes – such as the social, communal and corporate dimensions of this type of work, dealing as it does with communities.

We take capacity building to be a learning process with the goal of changing one or a mix of skills, knowledge, attitudes, or ways of thinking. Therefore, in this chapter, we will first briefly review a little of the vast literature on adult learning theory that has helped us understand in more depth how adults learn, which is primarily through and from experience. Following this, we will just as briefly visit the equally copious literature on the nature of art, to add to the throng another rarely discussed dimension: understanding art itself as learning experience. We have found that together, adult learning and art help us to explicate applied theatre training as an experiential learning process.

A messy procession

There is a general consensus about the 'messiness' of theorisations of adult learning. In the last four decades, multiple researchers, scholars, theorists, and practitioners have found it hard to organise the fragmenting, diversifying, and expanding field of adult education. Some writers talk about principles, theories, pedagogical procedure, assumptions, concepts, philosophy, and the characteristics of learners. Other scholars have been trying to organise the discussion around traditional learning theories, paradigms, and lenses. Standard existing theories, such as Malcolm Knowles's 'andragogical' model (1970), Jack Mezirow's 'transformative learning' (1991), and 'self-directed learning' (Knowles, 1975), are undergoing further development, new theories are gaining credence, with titles like 'embodied learning', 'somatic learning'

DOI: 10.4324/9781003426387-3

'neuroandragogy', and 'learning in the digital age'. Sometimes, different theories will cross-reference but frequently they do not build on each other. So, in researching and understanding adult learning, people are creating a kind of mosaic for it. There is no one-size-fits-all philosophy or theory. The choice of a paradigm or a perspective is a matter of which one best reflects the specific practice. Yi-Man decided to focus on '*experiential* learning' since applied theatre learning is, of course, experience-based.

Although there is an absence of consensus on adult learning, many scholars do agree 'experience' is its defining feature. Almost a century ago John Dewey laid a foundation for the role of experience in learning. Back in 1938 his classic book, *Experience and Education*, challenged the neglect by orthodox education of the personal experience of the learners. For him (and any intelligent observer today beyond the conventional school classroom), personal experience is a lifelong, continuous, and interactive part of human growth. Continuity and interaction in their active union with each other provide the measure of the educative significance and value of an experience. That can therefore provide the bedrock of adult learning, and becomes essential for adults (though Dewey would have seen it equally so for children). Adults have lived longer than children, have already built their own way of being in and seeing the world, others and themselves from past experiences.

Two camps

The most prominent adult learning theorists effectively group themselves into two camps: *Learning through reflection upon experience* and *Learning in experience*, what is known as the 'situated perspective'. We will just shake hands with a few of the most prominent adherents of the two camps.

Learning through reflection on experience

Dewey emphasises that reflective activity is a fundamental component of experiential learning. He stresses the difference between 'having' and 'knowing' an experience, For Dewey, reflective thought is the key to making it meaningful. Later followers of Dewey add more detail.

Kolb: the experiential learning cycle

David Kolb's theory (1984) describes how people with different learning styles learn by integrating their experiences with reflection. Learning is a tension- and conflict-filled process. Reflection is a cognitive process of analysis where experience is translated into concepts, which then turn out to be a guide for experimentation and the creation of further experience. Learners have to constantly choose which abilities should be used in a specific learning situation.

Boud: reflection in experiential learning

Similarly to Kolb, David Boud (Boud et al., 1985; Boud & Walker 1990) acknowledges that it is fundamentally through reflection that experience turns into learning, and he adds further enrichments. His model not only considers the impact of learning derived from the interaction between the context and the learner; but also recognises the role of feeling in the reflective process.

Both Kolb's and Boud's models give common concern to the learners' background and their prior learning capability. In addition, the mention of the role of feeling in Boud's model introduces some attention to the affective domain in the reflection process. However, the main focus of learning generated through experience is still very much reliant on cognitive processing.

Schön: reflective practice

Schön (1983, 1987) introduced his notion of reflective practice in the same period as the two models mentioned above. He also recognises the role of reflection playing a central role for learning to occur. Although his study is mainly focused on workplace learning, the applications are not limited to specific professions. Schön's ideas of learning through *reflection-on-* and *reflection-in-action* are commonly used in experiential learning beyond the workplace. Reflection-on- emphasises thinking about the experience after it has happened. In contrast, reflection-in- is taking place simultaneously while the practitioner is engaging in the experience. As we shall see throughout this book, those two distinct forms have now become an established part of applied theatre and classroom drama planning, and even within the dramatic activity itself (-in-action).

Situated learning

Applied theatre is a social art form. Its learning is fundamentally related to and influenced by the people involved and the place/context in which the learners are situated. Therefore, exploration of the understanding of experiential learning here is not limited to the individual dimension but involves the situated perspective. In contrast to the 'reflective' paradigm, whose main concern is on individual internal mental processes of learning, the situated perspective focuses on the socially interactive dimension of learning. Situated theorists perceive learning as the process of co-participation in the whole learning context, not just in the heads of individuals.

Wilson et al.: situated social learning

Arthur Wilson makes this point clearly:

> Adults no longer learn from experience, they learn in it, as they act in situations and are acted upon by situations.

(Wilson 1993: 75)

This view distinctly highlights the role of context, activity, and the importance of social interaction as the powerful place where learning occurs. Learning is also a process of enculturation where learners observe and practice *in situ* the behaviour of members of a culture, people pick up relevant jargon, imitate behaviour, and gradually start to act in accordance with its norms.

Lave and Wenger: communities of practice

All this implies that in situated cognition, learning is primarily embedded in doing. Situated learning theorists examine learning in communities and in practice. Drawing on their theory of 'communities of practice', Jean Lave and Etienne Wenger (1991) emphasise that learning, thinking, and knowing emerge through relations among people in activity in the socially and culturally structured world. The newcomer learns through social participation based on legitimate access to ongoing practice. Newcomers develop a changing understanding of practice, over a period of time, working with fellow community members who have different levels of knowledge and experience in the subject.

Fenwick: learning through embodiment

Tara Fenwick (2003) makes a clear claim that the moment of experiential learning occurs within action, with and among bodies. An embodied approach to experiential learning treats the sensual body as a site for learning instead of being a raw producer of data, where the mind still has the dominant role for generating knowledge. Experiential learning is unquestionably embodied in nature. The embodied view stresses we should not place all our emphasis on the rational, cognitive, and social mind at the expense of bodily competence as a way of knowing. In recognition of Michael Polanyi's concept of tacit knowledge (1958), embodied learning theorists see tacit/embodied/experiential knowing as the primal way of accessing knowledge. The knowing begins in the body before the learner can be consciously aware of it.

Holistic theories

From this cornucopia of partial insights presented by the followers of both camps have emerged some more integrated and holistic models. One of these Yi-Man eventually chose to use as her key analysis tool for understanding what was happening and had happened to the students in her workshops. To add to the occasional mentions of feeling and imagination by reflective and situated theorists, Heron considers them to be distinct from each other and both to be a vital part of learning through experience. He describes experiential learning as holistic in this significant sense that it integrates within the learning process perception, inner reactions such as emotion and imagination, outward action, and reflection.

Heron (1992) describes four ways of knowing – *experiential*, *presentational*, *propositional*, and *practical*. According to Heron, *experiential knowing* is the base and touchstone of the other three kinds of knowing. *Presentational knowing* arises from the encounter with experiential knowing. *Propositional knowing* is the traditional realm of 'knowledge about'. It is the intellectual knowing of ideas, of theory. *Practical knowing* is knowing how to do something. All four are interrelated with and built on each other.

We shall return to Heron's model later in the book (Chapter 9), because what distinguishes his model is the emphasis on feeling as a primary source of knowing; and he also recognises presentational knowing through a range of expressive art forms.

Making meaning from the mess

One may say that experiential learning scholarship is like the famous elephant and the blind philosophers. Cognitive and situated theorists alike touch parts of its features and try to define the whole. They highlight different areas of it for studying under their particular close lens, from either the individual or the social perspective.

Experiential learning is not an elephant. It has no fixed form. Learning experiences under different contexts, situations, and natures of practice are different in their shape. No one way to describe, interpret, and explain experiential learning can fully capture how the learning happens. We are still in the process of building our understanding of it. However, all these ideas are significant reference points that helped Yi-Man find out where applied theatre fits into the adult's essential learning experience.

Art as experience

So far, this review has been generalised, with nothing so uncerebral as real practice. Applied theatre as a kind of artistic experience also involves us in its distinct mode of aesthetic knowledge (which is addressed and defined below and in the next chapter).

In the past two decades, there has been a growing interest in the role of art in adult education literature. Increasing numbers of scholars recognise the contribution of the arts in facilitating effective adult learning in different contexts. However, most of the discussions are about the instrumental value of using art as a teaching medium, and often based on the hunches of trainers and practitioners. As yet, there has been little exploration of how the core theories of the arts themselves may be important. We now need to add another complementary dimension by briefly exploring a few of the widest-known art theories which relate art as an experience to the generation of learning and knowledge.

Drama and education

Artists themselves – especially dramatic ones – have always recognised and honoured the value and importance of their art as lifelong education, like the traditional Australian Aborigines, for whom seeing, hearing, and making art, performance, and learning are indivisible. For the Greek dramatists, art had various and sometimes conflicting educational aims. Euripides believed that virtue is teachable through the power of art, providing models of good for young people to follow all their lives. Plato feared it for the opposite reason, that those young people might follow the models of vice presented by the plays. More pragmatically, Aristotle analysed the constituents of dramatic art to find out what impact it has, seeking to identify – presciently for this book – both its intellectual and emotional effects.

Over two millennia on, twentieth-century followers of this didactic tradition, such as Brecht and a following generation of polemical dramatists, seized on the use of the dramatic aesthetic to get their audiences thinking, and so directly create real political action, on specific targets. Most followed Brecht in wanting to conscientise his audiences (which will be addressed In the next chapter). He was a passionate but impatient educationalist, making war on an audience's unthinking empathic identification with the story and characters that was typical of the illusionist theatre of his time – he was still thinking of artist and audience as separate entities, of course, a conventional assumption which the dramatic action in Yi-Man's research project drives a coach and horses through. Brecht's focus was all on replacing those emotional reactions with responses invoking conscious cognition. Later, both he and his followers in applied theatre and drama education learned some more sophisticated responses to the evocation and distancing of empathic emotion (Brecht's *verfremdungseffekt*, or alienation). Brechtian thinking became a cornerstone of contemporary theatre and drama education (eg Eriksson 2007), and it played a significant part in Yi-Man's training workshops. In contemporary theatre, particularly applied, and in drama education, the gap between the audience and the artist, with its aesthetic assumptions (the 'fourth wall'), has been problematised and often done away with, too.

Dewey again

Early in the twentieth century, Dewey, as we have seen, recognised the close interrelationship between art and learning, and instinctively the affective and social components of knowledge, and the importance of this integral relationship to lifelong learning. Since then, throughout the twentieth century thousands of eminent scholars from a range of art forms have studied the relationship. Because most of them, and the artists they study, come from the Western tradition of the individual artist, with the same accompanying binary distinction between the artist and the audience, the most famous have concentrated on analysing individual art-form expression, and its immediate effects on individual audience members. Each of them has contributed to identifying the aesthetic components of effective learning. For Yi-Man, two from the visual arts, and two more recent arts educators, provided key revelations and insights.

Susan Langer

Langer (1953) defines art as the creation of forms symbolic of human feeling. She further explains that art is not an actual feeling of the artist but a non-discursive symbol that expresses and projects the images of feeling. Art as an expressive form objectifies subjective feeling and makes it visible and perceivable for our contemplation and understanding. Deeply exploring the nature and function of symbolism, and being a visual arts specialist rather than from say drama or literature, she sets aside language, and makes a useful distinction between discursive and non-discursive symbolic expressions of mankind, broadening it to claim that the symbol-making function is the fundamental process of the human mind to formulate understanding. Discursive language cannot shape any extensive concepts of feeling. Since the inner life of any human being is 'nameless', we need other symbolic sources to express the subjective aspect of human experience. For Langer, art is the answer.

In Langer's theory of art, every work of art is an abstracted symbolisation of human feeling. Artists produce and sustain the symbol/illusion from the world of actuality and transform their motif into the works of art to create 'strangeness, separateness, other-ness' (1950: 519) for our contemplation, reflection, and understanding. The content of the significant form of art is a semblance that is opposite to the 'make-believe'. It is the 'make-*not*-believe' (1957: 42). The arts disengage us from the usual meanings we make of the familiar world by creating new images of reality. The normal forms are then 'freely conceived and composed in the interest of the artist's ultimate aim – significance, or logical expression' (1950: 519–520). Through the inward process of making an outward image, the works are made public as an objective symbol of the feeling, both to the makers and the others.

Louis Arnaud Reid

Like Langer, Reid stresses importance of the role of feeling in human experience and its crucial connection to the arts. He thinks it is a mistake to only validate propositional truth as knowledge and exclude the subjective aspects of knowing. For him, feeling is the immediate experience throughout conscious life working closely with thinking and action as the complex wholeness of the human organism.

Reid reminds us that feeling has a cognitive dimension to it. But it is not cognition that helps us to know; the 'cognitive-affective-feeling' is intrinsic and plays a vital part in knowing and understanding. He recognises art as a way of knowing, creating non-propositional aesthetic knowledge that calls on the holistic use of resources of the human being. The art-feelings are new and fresh in structure and specific to the meaning embodied in the artwork. (But beware, reader – see our comment about the meaning of 'meaning' below!) For Reid, the knowledge of art is a special kind of practical knowing-how that can be mainly guided by artistic or aesthetic intuition (1969: 215). We cannot 'talk *about* art' to learn, although the propositional talk can help the maker work more effectively in their next experience. He stresses we do art not by learning 'truths about' art, but 'on the job', by being involved in the art (1969: 216). The understanding knowledge of a work of art is genuinely shown in 'performing' practical competence. In recognition of the nature of immediacy in aesthetic experience, Reid, foreshadowing the situated theorists, suggests using the word 'embodiment' instead of 'expression'. He refers to aesthetic embodiment as something in active operation and the things expressed encounter 'a sea-change into something rich and strange'. Making art in the unknown is a discovery process that broadens our epistemology. What the artist discovers through making is not properly known till the making has been completed.

More than Langer, Reid turns his detailed attention to the experience of the audience as well as the art-maker. He usefully distinguishes two stages in coming to understand an artwork: the immediate experience of encountering the work, where the senses and feelings take the foreground as we 'apprehend' the work, then cognitive and critical awareness combine with them through time, distance and reflection as we come to 'comprehend' it (again, foreshadowing Schön).

Negotiability of meaning

Both Langer's and Reid's visions are very much focused on the individual artist and the symbolic expression and meaning-making that 'he' is making himself, and only secondarily on the audience, to whom is consigned the act of learning exactly **that** meaning from 'our contemplation, reflection and understanding'. It was a decade or two later that the radical philosophy of post-structuralism introduced the notion of meaning being jointly and actively constructed by the audience instead of them just being passive consumers of the artist's text. That was a contribution to this aesthetic discussion mainly from other art forms, notably literature and the reader-response theory of such as Stanley Fish and the new 'semiotics' (the study of signs and meanings) by – most famously – Roland Barthes, who shook the positivism of such as Langer with his – at the time shocking – title *The Death of the Author* (1967). Their shared discoveries of the co-construction of meaning between the author (and in education: teacher, curriculum) and the audience (students, learners) had an equally volcanic effect on education. It is now a vital tenet of constructivist education, too, and is one of the assumptions underlying this whole book. It will become plain in this book how important is the dismantling of the 'fourth wall' between transmitters and receivers in both education and dramatic art. Applied theatre too is developing structures, strategies and techniques to activate the audience and turn them into working participants in an aesthetically driven learning experience.

Elliott Eisner and connoisseurship

By the end of the twentieth century, a couple of generations of scholarship later, the two fields or art and education cohere and are eloquently united in what is (at least in the arts education world) a largely accepted fusion of art and learning. This is expressed by contemporaries such as Elliot Eisner, a widely respected and still current philosopher of both education and the arts – so, Dewey's successor, as a scholar who understood both fields deeply in theory and practice. Both he and Dewey recognised the indissoluble interconnection between arts and learning. Eisner spoke firmly of the 'art of education', and describes the kinship between them. He insisted that anyone seeking to understand, critique, or change either of them must have a 'connoisseurship' in both. He claims that the arts provide conditions for us to notice the world around us and the nuances in it. They bring a new way of knowing through reading images, and train habits of mind to be aware of things originally experienced unconsciously. Working in the arts involves tolerating ambiguity and suspending judgement based on set rules. Something new is nurtured from the unknown. It brings us fresh perspectives to perceive and interpret the world of understanding. The arts as expressive form often generate empathic feeling that makes action happen. To empathise with others is a kind of ability to understand others' experience and a root of compassion. Indeed, the arts closely connect with our subjective life. Working in the arts can give us the means to look inward to what we feel and believe, to discover our inner emotional selves: in Eisner's (2002) words, exploring our interior landscape. And also in the process of creation, the arts can be a vehicle to turn our internal self into the visible works which allow us to inspect our own thinking. He emphasises that learning in the arts is a way of enriching our awareness and expanding our humanity (2008).

Winston and beauty

To close this visit to the world of theory, we will include the refreshing moral vision of beauty from Joe Winston, unconsidered by other scholars in the field of adult education and understandably barely heard-of (originally an early-childhood teacher, and, significantly, primarily a drama educator too). He shares Eisner's emphasis on the importance to humanity of the aesthetic experience. But Winston (2010) puts his core concern more broadly, boldly using a word unthinkable in conventional education settings, and even quite unfashionable in art: that *beauty* is a fundamental human need. He quotes Arthur Danto, 'Beauty is an option for art…But it is not an option for life' (2008: 80). Nevertheless, the value of beauty is still the central concern of art. Reclaiming beauty as a potential force for learning and for good, Winston argues 'beauty is powerfully formative and intrinsically associated with virtue' (2008: 72).

Winston stresses that, providing energy for good action, the soft values (like love, sympathy, trust, gentleness, etc.) will be found in beauty with life-enhancing qualities. Values create motivational force to support continuing learning through the aesthetic experience. We gain knowledge through practice driven by our desires shaped by beauty. This is 'real knowledge' underpinned by the sense of values that Winston maintains it is necessary to create and express in the purposeful artistic experience.

Implications of art for adult learning

Learning in the arts reminds us that feeling is one of the important aspects of human knowing. It is tacit in nature but irreplaceable in creating human understanding from experience. This aesthetic domain of knowing has been little explored and largely overlooked by the adult experiential learning theorists of either constructivist reflective or situated paradigms. For the constructivists who see experiential learning as a conscious mental activity, knowledge is generated through reflective thought in and on action. Although they do mention the senses and feeling in the learning process, these aspects are either one of the learning styles to grasp experience (like Kolb) or a complementary element to assist effective reflection (like Boud et al.). Deep study of the arts tells us that affective knowing in experience plays more than this merely supporting role. As Louis Arnaud Reid stresses, cognitive and affective knowing are inseparable. When we define learning from experience, we cannot neglect feeling as an integral part of knowing. The human mind functions in a coherent system without splitting cognition and sensation, but working together.

References

Boud, D., Keogh, R., & Walker, D. (Eds.). (1985). *Reflection: Turning experience into learning.* London: Kogan Page Ltd.

Boud, D., & Walker, D. (1990). Making the most of experience. *Studies in Continuing Education, 12*(2), 61–80.

Dewey, J. (1938). *Experience and education.* New York: Macmillan.

Eisner, E. W. (2002). *The arts and the creation of mind.* New Haven: Yale University Press.

Eisner, E. W. (2008). Art and knowledge. In J. G. Knowles, & A. L. Cole, (Ed.), *Handbook of the arts in qualitative research: Perspectives, methodologies, examples, and issues* (pp. 3–12). Thousand Oaks: SAGE.

Eriksson, S. A. (2007). Distance and awareness of fiction: Exploring the concepts. *NJ – National Journal of Drama Australia, 31*(1), 5–22.

Fenwick, T. (2003). Reclaiming and re-embodying experiential learning through complexity science. *Studies in the Education of Adults, 35*(2), 123–141.

Heron, J. (1992). *Feeling and personhood: Psychology in another key.* London: SAGE.

Knowles, M. S. (1970). *The modern practice of adult education; andragogy versus pedagogy.* New York: Association Press.

Knowles, M. S. (1975). *Self-directed learning: A guide for learners and teachers.* Englewood Cliffs, NJ: Cambridge Adult Education.

Kolb, D. A. (1984). *Experiential Learning: Experience as the source of learning and development.* Englewood Cliffs, NJ: Prentice-Hall.

Langer, S. K. (1950). The principles of creation in art. *The Hudson Review, 2*(4), 515–534.

Langer, S. K. (1953). *Feeling and form: A theory of art developed from philosophy in a new key.* New York: Charles Scribner & Sons.

Langer, S. K. (1957). *Problems of art.* New York: Charles Scribner & Sons.

Lave, J., & Wenger, E. (1991). *Situated learning: Legitimate peripheral participation.* Cambridge, UK: Cambridge University Press.

Mezirow, J. (1991). *Transformative dimensions of adult learning.* San Francisco: Jossey-Bass.

Polanyi, M. (1958). *Personal knowledge: Towards a post-critical philosophy.* London: Routledge & Kegan Paul.

Reid, L. A. (1969). *Meaning in the arts.* London: George Allen & Unwin Ltd.

Schön, D. A. (1983). *The reflective practitioner: How professionals think in action.* New York: Basic Books.

Schön, D. A. (1987). *Educating the reflective practitioner.* San Francisco: Jossey-Bass.

Wilson, A. (1993). The promise of situated cognition. *New Directions in Adult and Continuing Education, 57,* (pp. 71–79) Retrieved from https://doi.org/10.1002/ace.36719935709

Winston, J. (2010). *Beauty and education. Routledge international studies in the philosophy of education (24).* New York, London: Routledge.

3 Dramatic learning

Preamble

In the previous chapter, we began to explore how adults learn best through experience and we touched on the concept of art itself as a learning experience. Now it is time to focus on applied theatre, its central principles, and its relationship to drama education. This will take us to the particular forms of applied theatre that Yi-Man chose for the participants' experiences in her training workshop and begin to identify those theatrical and pedagogical experiences which played the most important roles in their learning journey.

Applied theatre – what is it?

Applied theatre is a term that has been gaining currency since it was coined in the last decade of the twentieth century. Applied theatre emerged as a definable and distinct practice along with its established literature, principles, and practice from two complementary and overlapping parent movements. The first of these, growing throughout the twentieth century, involved the regular use of drama in school classrooms as a learning tool, earlier known as *drama-in-education* (DiE) and more commonly now just *drama education* (DE) or *educational drama* (the reasons for the change of nomenclature will be seen later this chapter). The other movement, *theatre for development* (TfD), emerged in the second half of the century, mainly comprising theatre professionals working with adults and in communities for specific purposes other than entertainment – usually either directly political or instrumental to community development. There is more-or-less consensus now about the specific usage of the term, and a growing literature and body of established practice.

In the Chinese context it is a matter of translation, with the words for 'drama' and 'theatre' used more or less interchangeably. Throughout this book we are also using drama and theatre mostly interchangeably. Which term is used depends on the objectives and contexts of their applications – with the word theatre usually indicating some kind of formal performance.

There is now a general understanding of applied theatre as an umbrella or collective term to describe *theatre practices and performative activities applied*

DOI: 10.4324/9781003426387-4

to educational, institutional, and community contexts, with a primary purpose other than entertainment. Its common features are:

- It takes place not in traditional theatre venues, but in a variety of social, institutional, and informal settings;
- The audience, who may or may not have drama experience or skills, is in some way actively involved in the process, and applied theatre makers often prefer the term 'participants' to 'audiences' or 'students';
- The work that is created and/or performed arises from the concerns and issues of the specific audience/participant group, or their sponsors;
- Its aims are either to serve personal, social, or community change, or specific vocational training.

As an umbrella term, applied theatre therefore can be seen to subsume both its parent movements, drama education and TfD. Many teachers in schools still prefer one of the educational terms, though TfD is less often used world-wide nowadays. I should note that these definitions are not tablets of stone, and recent innovations within 'mainstream theatre' constantly produce creative slippage and porous borders, as Peter O'Connor points out:

> Many theatre companies increasingly engage in more socially committed and participatory forms of theatre, perhaps most spectacularly realized in the enormously popular forms of immersive theatre that now span days of improvised politically charged events attended by tens of thousands of people.
>
> (2022, 71)

'But is it art?'

From the early days, there was widespread concern that the instrumental primary purposes of applied theatre would diminish its aesthetic power. In the first edition of the *Applied Theatre Researcher* (2001/2022) Björn Rasmussen discusses:

> …to what extent the cultural contexts change the aesthetic approaches. At one end of the continuum, you have dramatic applications that are context-related to such an extent that they have lost their aesthetic power and autonomy.

This concern added to a fierce debate that had already been going on about drama in schools, especially in the UK. This was led by attacks on the participatory form of drama then known as DiE, now known as 'process drama', by adherents of education in traditional dramatic art, such as David Hornbrook (1989), who pointed out with asperity the poor artistic quality of much of the early process drama work. This did indeed focus on its pedagogical purposes, some of it was aesthetically weak, and its own rather different and quite new processual aesthetic was not yet properly recognised or cared for, even by its strongest proponents. A similar attack on theatre-in-education (TiE) – the parallel use of participatory professional theatre in schools, often with significant audience participation – was witheringly articulated in 1988 by Australian playwright Alex Buzo: 'The TiE people do a great job educating children, but it's not art, and it's not entertainment' (quoted in O'Toole 2009: 164). This carried the debate into the burgeoning world of applied theatre, backed up by critics from the world of TfD, such as Jamil Ahmed (2002), who pointed out TfD's frequent ineffectuality and poor value for money for either its beneficiaries or its sponsors, in many well-meaning developmental contexts.

This two-pronged attack had two valuable effects: scholars of both process drama and TiE sprang to their defence, energetically defining what the new aesthetic configuration and re-imagined artistic components of process actually were, with titles like 'An aesthetic framework for drama: issues and implications' (McLean 1996) and 'Aesthetic engagement in the drama process' (Bundy 2003). Ever since, practitioners right across the fields have paid a great deal more attention to the aesthetic component in our work – and it is central to this book.

A 'new' aesthetic?

In the second half of the twentieth century, as we indicated in Chapter 2, theatre workers and schoolteachers both started to dismantle the 'fourth wall' between the actors and the audience – each group frequently influenced by Brecht's crusade to directly influence audiences into action for social change.

Part of this change involved the growing innovation and use of spontaneous forms of drama, mainly types of improvisation. The dramatic action or performance is not pre-scripted. Improvised drama requires the participants to act in the immediate given circumstances in any drama, in role. They have to think on their feet, make spontaneous decisions, and respond to the unexpected in a flexible, creative way. The result of the drama is often unknown and always open to possibilities. '… about journeys and not knowing how the journeys may end' (Heathcote, in O'Neill, 2015: 53). In this participatory form of drama, people involved are always working in a process of becoming.

This innovation and shift in drama was to be enormously influenced by a rapidly growing systematic study of young children's spontaneous social dramatic play. Early scholars who analysed this, such as Peter Slade (1956), noticed that the whole dramatic experience is negotiated by the children among themselves as they go along. There are rules and structures, both physical, spatial, and dramatic, to which the players adhere, and which somehow they know – if not, the play falls apart and stops – but while the children observe them a coherent narrative emerges, and sometimes multiple progressive narratives, peopled by consistent characters. Like any grown-up drama, all these are sustained by tension, emotional absorption, and total collaboration of all participants. In other words, as Slade proclaimed, they have their own distinct aesthetic form.

This early scholarship and growing observation and analysis were enthusiastically seized on by a movement of schoolteachers and early childhood scholars, some with professional knowledge of drama. They saw that it might be applied in formal classrooms with older children – later, even adults. The movement originated mainly in the United Kingdom, where it became known as drama-in-education and was enthusiastically spread round the globe by its adherents. They were much attracted by its characteristics of spontaneity, group negotiation in the moment and natural empathic identification of the players with the characters they were creating. This seemed to offer a practical, dramatic way to fulfil the ideals of creative, dialogic and open education presaged by the constructivist educators from Dewey onward, whom we met in Chapter 2.

Experimentation with children's play gathered pace; early practitioners gradually formalised it so that it would be manageable within classrooms. They also melded it with other improvised dramatic activities, such as rehearsal games and participatory techniques that were contemporaneously being invented by the closely kindred theatre-in-education movement, such as 'teacher-in-role', participant 'enrolment' and flexible narrative structures, all of which we shall meet in Yi-Man's project. Gradually, a distinct and recognisable new genre of drama took shape. It is still based on the spontaneity and social negotiability of children's play, but with a leader or teacher controlling a more formal dramatic structure with a clear educational purpose – whether initially suggested by the students or by the leader – and adhering to the constraints of schools' teaching spaces and timetables. In all these senses it is processual and has no pre-conceived outcome or performance product – it exists experientially in the moment for the participants. So, from around 1990, it acquired its own nomenclature: 'process drama', a title by which it is now almost universally known, which superseded the more ambiguous 'drama-in-education' originally used to denote equally either process drama or any other classroom-based dramatic activity.

Its participants may have no clear-cut role as either actor or spectator. In process drama, the participants play multiple roles of playwright, director, dramaturge, actor, and audience, sometimes several simultaneously. Jonothan Neelands sharply explicates this feature:

> All present are assumed to be 'players' as well as spectators of their own and others' acting in response to the demands of the imagined world. It is not a form of drama in which it is assumed that only some of us can act whilst the rest can only watch and react. It is a direct rather than directed form of drama that requires social and artistic acting together in order to create imagined worlds and events. Without the social and artistic actions of those present, nothing happens and nothing is made.
>
> (2011: 170)

It occurs to us that the renegotiation of dramatic meaning that this revolutionary dismantling of the fourth wall symbolised something akin to the 'death of the author' and reader-response theory (they were, in fact, more or less contemporaneous, too). Add to that, because it is drama, not literature, it is of course live, first-hand experience for all participants, and not just the designated actors. At times, they all take the roles of an internal audience – it's just there are no external spectators, as the experience itself is the learning.

More broadly across the applied theatre scene, that does not mean that the concepts of the actor and performance had suddenly disappeared. Actors (people who imagine and interact) are at the heart of all forms of theatre/drama. They use the dramatic elements to create an 'as-if' world which suspends belief from the real world to convey aesthetic meaning. In order to pretend, they need to work with their imaginative capacity. Through the dramatic action, the image in mind is externalised and expressed in the aesthetic space. In process drama, they are the participants themselves.

Liberatory theatre for change

Dorothy Heathcote and her process drama has been influential in the development of applied theatre, because her experiential drama has the declared purpose not of entertainment, but of personal and societal change, which is always one of the primary drivers of applied theatre.

> The most important manifestation about this thing called drama is that it must show change. It does not freeze a moment in time, it freezes a problem in time, and you examine the problem as the people go through a process of change.
>
> (Heathcote, in Prentki & Preston, 2009: 200)

Around the same time, on the other side of the globe in Brazil, and even more influential for applied theatre, another revolutionary theatre pioneer, Augusto Boal, started the first of his several liberatory theatre movements: 'Theatre of the oppressed' (TO). Both pioneers were largely driven by the same key theorists – educationalists Paolo Freire [1972/2012] and Lev Vygotsky [1957/2014], and, from theatre, Bertold Brecht. Freire's central concept of education as '*Conscientizacao*', a developmental process of social consciousness-raising, became Boal's goal and watchword.

Heathcote and Boal had basically the same aims, but they had opposite dramatic starting points and pedagogical settings. Boal was working not in schools but in a professional political community theatre in the poorest areas of Brazil, such as the favelas of Rio, seeking to help the inhabitants to overcome their social and personal oppressions. He and his company worked out that *conscientizacao* could be generated through workshops of actors' exercises, and a participatory style of performance he called 'forum theatre', where the audiences are presented with short, improvised plays based on a scene of oppression, sometimes their own, and invited as 'spect-actors' to intervene in the play to suggest ways of overcoming the oppression.

The actor and the real world

Through the lens of this new aesthetic, it becomes clearer how emotion works to assist learning towards change for participants in any theatre, but particularly the new improvisatory forms.

> To take on a role is to detach oneself from what is implicitly understood and to blur temporarily the edges of a given world. It invites modification, adjustment, reshaping, and realignment of concepts already held. Through detachment from experiencing one can look at one's experiencing anew.
>
> (Bolton, 1985: 156)

This embodied existence through a special act of imagination brings actors and audience and/or participants to engage with what is going on, by holding both the real and the fictional world in mind at the same time – as Gavin Bolton, one of Heathcote's collaborators, puts it: 'they are in dual consciousness' (1984: 141). He also analyses how the embodied imaginative act generates emotion for learning in the same way, through what visionary Russian educational philosopher Lev Vygotsky similarly names 'dual affect: the child weeps in play as a patient, but revels as a player' (in Bolton, 1984: 106). Bolton points out that drama requires the participants to work with emotional engagement to make meaning. They may identify their own disposition with the characters' emotion as a mental projection for raising self-awareness.

Heightened awareness is also one of the key characteristics of aesthetic engagement, as it is defined by Bundy (2003). In her research, she indicates that animation, connection, and heightened awareness are the keys to aesthetic experience. Through animation, participants become more alive and more alert to themselves and the world around them. The drama works only if they engage with the idea, at a metaphorical level. The idea can connect to the associations which participants make, that link the fictional context to their real-world existence. The potential for new knowledge emerging will occur as drama provides opportunities to see things in a new light and possibly leads to change.

Reflection is also essential in all forms of applied theatre for helping participants to synthesise and consolidate the experience. Heathcote emphasises, 'without reflection there is no learning from the experience' (Johnson & O'Neill 1984: 209). Reflection can occur either during a period of collective discussion about the dramatic experience or perhaps while participants are engaged in thinking, speaking, writing, reading, or drawing, and even while doing the drama itself. In 'as-if' dramatic contexts, participants are free to examine a multitude of meanings as well as reflect on them through action. Reflection in applied theatre is not purely a mental activity; it is visualised, articulated, and shared. Knowing can become more tangible and concrete for further exploration. Drama is an art form oriented in the concrete experience of action and reflection – imagining through concrete action, recollecting, hypothesising, re-creating, and musing.

The activities used in applied theatre training are flexible and diverse. It incorporates various types of experience by providing new physical routines (in games and exercises), new action resources (the acting of unfamiliar characters in new locations), and the experience of reworking a range of dramatic action (through participation in theatrical rehearsal, improvisation or performance) for the participants. These experiences emerge from the hidden textures of participants' bodies as they perform, as well as leaving traces on those bodies.

Applied theatre involves not only individual action but also the interconnected actions of participants. Participants can be marked by the conduct of others. They express and externalise their thoughts and images in mind. They see the alternative actions and responses from others. They may take this as their own reference, imitate it, or copy it. Furthermore, they can gain more self-understanding when they see themselves in others' responses. Individual differences will be channelled into collective actions. Ultimately, it is what the individual draws from the collective meanings that matters; they find part of 'I' as well as the 'Not I' through their interaction.

In addition to this social interactive process, there are other important qualities which are a by-product of the dramatic experience, like concentration, trust, sensitivity, cooperation, patience, tolerance, confidence, respect, perception, judgement, social concern, coping with ambivalent feelings, empathy, and responsibility. These attributes foster individual change. A sense of self-advancement reinforces personal growth. An increasing self-efficacy helps participants to have a feeling of competency to adopt change. Change is not a promise in applied theatre, but it does create the potential and foundation for human change, or as a first step, for 'change of understanding' (Bolton, 1984: 153).

Yi-Man's three chosen genres

Applied theatre practice has many genres, and each individual approach has its specific philosophy and tradition for its strategies and activities. Some aim at creating performance with or for the participants; others merely focus on the interaction among participants in the dramatic action, where no theatrical output is necessary. Yi-Man chose three different genres in the training workshop, based on her own understanding of their potential application in Chinese NGOs, according to her previous field experience. She also chose to diversify the strategies introduced in the training so that participants would have more variety of choice for their own uses. Apart from the common factor of the potential for human change through applied theatre discussed above, the three genres included in the training workshop also have their own aesthetic pattern in the creation of their artwork, and particular features for facilitating change.

> The theatre of the oppressed is a system of physical exercises, aesthetic games, image techniques and special improvisations whose goal is to safeguard, develop and reshape this human vocation, by turning the practice of theatre into an effective tool for the comprehension of social and personal problems and the search for their solutions.
>
> (Boal, 1995: 14–15)

> Theatre of the oppressed (TO) has two fundamental linked principles: it aims (a) to help the spect-actor transform himself into a protagonist of the dramatic action and rehearse alternatives for his situation, so that he may then be able (b) to extrapolate into his real life the actions he has rehearsed in the practice of theatre.
>
> (Boal, 1995: 40)

Augusto Boal created and worked in this particular kind of applied theatre from the 1970s onward, and his work still has many followers and adherents, in 'pure' or modified forms. The heart of his performance work is to break down the passivity of the spectators, for them to become 'spect-actors', transforming the act in theatre into action in real life. He asserts that 'theatre is the capacity that all of us have, as human beings, to observe ourselves in action' (1996: 47). The ability for self-observation is a language we already possess. TO was created to help people develop the capacity to use this language better.

Boal calls this characteristic of drama, which allows participants to hold two worlds in mind at the same time, 'metaxis'. TO puts it at the centre of its practice. Participants interplay between 'the image of the reality' and 'the reality of the image' (1995: 43). This corresponds with Bolton's 'dual affect'. Playing with the embodied image in the fictional world is similarly the essence of the image theatre Boal promoted. The imagination and experimental thoughts disrupt the taken-for-granted world; the possible self, others, and reality emerge-in-action for the participants to learn something previously unknown. Theatre provides an aesthetic space where things are more plastic, more contrasting, and magnified. Time and space can be condensed or stretched at will; memory and imagination can be liberated: we are not only ourselves, but also the actors and the characters – the subjects who tell the story as well as the objects to whom the things have happened. Therefore, this aesthetic space creates a powerful platform to look into our situation and to analyse it. A systematisation of exercises (physical monologues), games (physical dialogues), and techniques of image theatre and forum theatre, which are the arsenal of TO, can serve for all of us the purpose of development of the capacity to express ourselves through theatre.

TO participants usually bring as starting materials their lives, feelings, stories, experiences, and experiences of oppression, and this includes personal values and beliefs. They will directly expose themselves and their thinking within the group and explore the ideas from a shared understanding and collective learning. One story becomes 'our' story. The participants can see through to the systems that lie behind the scene, and develop a new understanding, new knowledge, and, more importantly, become 'actors' in life. Potential change occurs in TO, based on participants' discovery and reflection. Learning something new gives alternatives and more choices in life; this knowledge can change participants who might also change the people around them.

Process drama

The current central understanding and principles of process drama are still indebted to the two most influential historical figures in the field, Dorothy Heathcote and Gavin Bolton, who provided insights into drama as an effective medium of human learning. In the experience of emotional engagement and the release of imagination through the lived-through process, drama creates a cognitive/affective learning potential for gaining new insight and understanding. According to leading practitioner and writer of process drama (in theory and practice) Cecily O'Neill (1995: 12–13), the key characteristics of process drama include that it: generates a fictional world which will be inhabited for the insights, interpretations, and understanding it may yield; is based on a powerful 'pre-text'; is built up from a series of episodes which are both improvised and composed or rehearsed; takes place over a timespan; involves the whole group in the same enterprise; and has no external spectators, but participants are an audience for their own actions. 'Pre-text' is a word that O'Neill coined and has become common usage to describe 'the source or impulse for the drama process' (1995:xv). It launches the first moment of the action, establishing location, atmosphere, roles, and situations within the drama. It gives an invitation to the participants to enter into the context and involve themselves in active role-taking. All participants need to agree to suspend their disbelief and temporarily accept an illusion, to co-create a fictitious world with the facilitator and together to interrogate and transform ideas, values, attitudes, and visions within the world.

A process drama is not necessarily in the form of linear narrative, as the aim is not just to tell a story, but to identify and explore in depth important moments within a narrative, to piece together a group understanding of the significance of the story. It is therefore constructed in a number of different segments by interweaving spontaneous 'living-through role-play' with dramatic 'conventions' (Neelands & Goode, 2000) and theatrical and rehearsal techniques. The episodic structure allows the gradual articulation of a complex dramatic world and enables it to be extended and elaborated through different frames. The whole group will be engaged in the same encounter collectively, to examine an event and crystallise the layers of meaning.

Unlike other applied theatre genres in which reflection is always organised after the dramatic scene or experience, in process drama reflection can take place both in-role and out-of-the-role, within and beyond the drama. Participants in process drama, shifting their mindsets to play with different identities, are allowed to reflect within the immediate interactive experience and act on their reflection at the same time. This engagement of the affective, critical, metacognitive, and creative thinking embodied in the dramatic event potentially develops their capacity for higher order thinking.

A typical strategy of process drama is 'Teacher-in-Role' (TiR), which also makes this genre different from others. The facilitator or leader in process drama will frequently enter the fiction and interact with the participants in role to deepen their response and commitment. The use of this strategy will alter the teaching and learning relationship by shifting the leader's power and status (the one who knows and owns the knowledge and the dramatic structure). Participants are co-authors in creating the drama: they can be empowered to go beyond their normal roles and develop their agency, for instance by the leader taking the role of a low-status, humble or information-seeking character: ceding the power so that the participants can take over and progress the drama. This is something that rarely happens in classrooms, school or adult!

Unlike in TO, participants in process drama will not ask nor be asked to play themselves and use their real-life stories to create drama. In process drama, experiencing and then coming back from a fictional dramatic world, the characters, situations, events and issues within the world are like a refracting mirror to newly illuminate the real world.

Participatory theatre

The third phase of Yi-Man's workshop is not strictly a single genre, but a conglomeration of domains of applied theatre which place the art of public performance as the major element in the practice. These include genres such as theatre-in-education, forum theatre, outreach theatre, prison theatre, museum and other location theatre, community theatre, theatre for development and agit-prop. Though they may have different structures and locations, agendas, rationales, and target audiences, to a certain extent they do share similar social, educational, and interventionist goals for change. All of them also share the characteristic of including a measure of live audience participation, to engage their audiences mentally and physically, breaking the fabled fourth wall at least a bit, and sometimes completely.

Participation

There is a wide spectrum of participatory formats in this genre. Back in 1976, co-author John O'Toole categorised three types of participation based on his observations of UK theatre-in-education:

Extrinsic, where the element of participation is separated from the theatricality, by a workshop or audience discussion;

Peripheral, where the audience is invited to contribute to add to the theatricality without affecting either the structure and nature of the play or their spectators' role as an audience.

Integral, where the audience perspective becomes the perspective of characters within the drama, especially when the audience members act as well as being acted upon.

(88)

Anthony Jackson adds forum theatre to the list to differentiate this form of participatory theatre which has 'a very specific set of goals and working methods…and distinctive in its encouragement of the audience (as "spect-actors") to influence the outcomes of the drama' (2011: 236).

TiE teams bring learner-centred pedagogy into schools 'through participatory practices which were devised from a starting-point in the lives of the children' (Prentki, 1998:484). Diverse strategies have been developed to break from the normal routine of traditional theatre, where the audience can be actively involved, taking part in the whole performance emotionally as well as physically, just as in process drama. As in process drama – which shares many of its early UK progenitors with TiE – these 'living-through' experiences can have distancing moments and techniques built-in, where the participants can recognise themselves in the situation or factual story from which the TiE programme (as they are usually called) was created.

Actors in this form will usually have an additional function beyond that of performers, and early on they were christened 'actor-teachers'. They take up the functions of teachers or facilitators in the meaning-making process as they research and design the learning journey by incorporating interactive strategies; they also facilitate the whole process often from within their roles as characters in the drama. This was where the 'teacher-in-role' strategy originated.

There is an obvious overlap with forum theatre (one of the major strategies used in the later stages of theatre of the oppressed) where audience members are encouraged to intervene in the rehearsed or improvised drama at a crisis point to give advice to the characters in order to find out possible solutions for the issues being performed. Boal observes the development of this form has been 'a constant search for dialogical forms, forms of theatre through which it is possible to converse' (cited in Jackson, 2007: 183) with the audience. Facilitators in forum theatre, whom Boal dubbed 'jokers', are usually not acting members. They take the position of a direct link between the audience (the real world) and the dramatic action (the fictional world); their role is also to motivate and enable the audience to practise their power to intervene, to act. In theatre-in-education with integral participation, the participants' interaction is usually not so transient and temporary as the interventions in forum theatre – it lasts throughout the whole performance.

Creating a space for dialogue, which in a broad sense is a major aim of both TiE and forum theatre, is activated by the theatre piece. It can happen when the audience is directly engaged in the discussion of the problems in the drama, seeking their resolution. Once this happens, the embodied voices released are diverse, which stimulates further conflicts of thought, leading to further debate and also critical reflection. Jackson (2005, 2007) stresses the power to sustain and enrich the dialogue of the aesthetic, working interdependently with the instrumental, that is at work in participatory theatre. The performance (that is, the theatrical performance) is the crucible in which existing dialogues are opened up – brought into a particular, heightened, and sharpened focus – and new dialogues are added: dialogues between actors and audience; author (the text) and audience; characters and characters; and characters and audience-in-role (as in TiE and forum) (Jackson 2007: 187).

It is worth clarifying here the distinction between *audience participation* in the play or performance itself, which is what is referred to here, and common to both TiE and forum theatre, and *community participation* in theatre. There is another kind of participatory theatre which does not rely on the audience–performer interaction format nor alter the orthodox separation of performers from audience. This is most usually found in TfD, community theatre, and youth theatre. Participants are not audience but artists, actively engaged in the theatre-making process, working along with the applied theatre practitioners usually to make a public performance. Marcia Pompêo-Nogueira (2002) argues that this kind of theatre 'appears to be the most esteemed contemporary theatre for development' in her own context of Brazilian community theatre.

> Theatre *by* the people represents a process that involves the community throughout the process, including the making of the drama, which is based on themselves and their problem. Here the community is asked to be involved from the identification of the problem until the final performance.
>
> (107)

The practice is based on a perspective that theatre is for everyone, and it can be made by any group of people. Participants are not passive recipients; through artistic production, they can voice their concerns, do their own thinking, and present their own views. Participants share stories, and then refine, reshape, and rehearse them to re-present them to external audiences with the help of a professional theatre maker, who acts as the co-deviser.

> This is a dialectical process of reclaiming ownership and autonomy…it begins the process of conscientisation, through imagination and creativity, that may lead to a people-centred practice of self-development.
>
> (Pammenter, 2013: 94–95)

To understand the democratisation of the creating process in this kind of theatre, Christine Sinclair developed a community theatre matrix 'as a way of understanding the evolution and development of a community theatre event' (2006: 36). 'The Engaged Space' is a crucial organising principle for her model.

She proposes agency, pedagogy, artistry, pragmatics and critical reflection to be the key elements contributing to the collective art-making process, and that community theatre practitioners should be aware of these.

> Engaged Space can encompass a wide range of interactions and a diversity of inputs and can accommodate the artistic and the social, the pedagogic and the therapeutic and also, and sometimes most importantly, the practical.
>
> (2006: 44)

The possibility of community enactment and change will evolve beyond the space of participatory theatre, perhaps leading to eventual social transformation within the community.

The applied theatre training workshop

In Yi-Man's study, the people involved are not merely participants coming to experience applied theatre; they also have a clear agenda to learn how to use its multiple contexts

In *The Process of Drama* (1992), John O'Toole explores in depth the four different contexts that are at play and being negotiated in the process of creating any drama:

- The real context – the background, prior experience, interests, and beliefs brought by each individual participant, and their shared experiences.
- The context of the setting – the particular place and space where the drama takes place.
- The context of the medium – the coming together of the participant group.
- The fictional context – the world created within the drama.

Apart from the fictional context, which is what happens within the dramatic fiction, the other three represent the external world outside the drama. As we have suggested, the collision of the real contexts of the participants with the fictional context within the dramatic process is where meaning is created, and that provides the impact for generating change in understanding.

However, in Yi-Man's training workshop, the real context is not only the consciousness of the 'luggage' of their prior experiences that participants bring with them, to be managed as a bridge to a fictional context. It also plays an independent role as a space for the trainee learners to consolidate, coordinate, and connect their learning experiences. In an applied theatre training workshop involving three different genres, for example, a fictional context will not be created in every session. The participants will spend a relatively longer time in the real context – the training workshop (the context of the setting). Borrowing a definition from Richard Schechner (2002: 198–199), training is a process where specific skills are learned and practised. Workshop is a process where materials are found, invented, and played with. In training, learners acquire techniques through practice in the craft, an organic training where the learning is by immersion and imitation and not rigid. Learners should discover their own 'new' both in the fictional context and in the real contexts.

In a workshop the social interaction becomes more complex and multi-layered. In the real context outside the drama, the participants will bring and deal with not only their relationships but also their personal agendas and collective learning objectives. In the fictional context, they don't just bring themselves in to interact with the contents and materials; they will also need to remain distanced enough to observe how the methods are being operated and being managed. Therefore, the contexts of the setting and medium of the training workshop are crucial elements for facilitating learning through the active and reciprocal engagement of participants.

An important aspect of Yi-Man's hypotheses underlying this project were that the pedagogical experience in the workshop would create a new relationship between the people, the space, and the art form. This inside-out learning approach would bring the participants new language to express themselves through artistic and aesthetic means. In the learning space, they and their thinking would be visible and shared, which could foreshadow new possibilities or new understanding.

Segue

In these last two chapters we have identified what we know and understand about both adult education and applied theatre, which combined to provide the basis for Yi-Man's unusual and lengthy training workshop. Would it fulfil all the ideals of adult education and applied theatre? The proof of the pudding would be in the eating, for the participants, and for their facilitator too.

So, for the next four chapters we are inviting you to share their thoughts and deep considerations about the meal. For that we shall return our address to the first person, as Yi-Man not only takes again up her story of the workshop, but also selects the choicest and richest of the participants' responses, to lay before the reader: inviting you to share their thoughts about the applied theatre learning they gained, the other equally important generic learnings they gained, and about Yi-Man herself!

References

Ahmed, S. J. (2002). Wishing for a World without 'Theatre for Development': Demystifying the case of Bangladesh. *Research in Drama Education: The Journal of Applied Theatre and Performance, 7*(2), 207–219.

Boal, A. (1995). *The rainbow of desire: The Boal method of theatre and therapy.* London: Routledge.

Boal, A. (1996). Politics, education and change. In J. O'Toole & K. Donelan (Eds.), *Drama, culture and empowerment: the IDEA dialogues* (pp. 47–52) Brisbane: IDEA Publications.

Bolton, G. (1984). *Drama as education*. London: Longman.

Bolton, G. (1985). Changes in thinking about Drama in Education. *Theory into Practice, 24*(3), 151–157.

Bundy, P. (2003). Aesthetic engagement in the drama process. *Research in Drama Education, 8*(2), 171–181.

Freire, P. (1972/2012). *Pedagogy of the oppressed*. New York: Bloomsbury.

Heathcote, D. (2009). Drama as a process for change. In T. Prentki & S. Preston (Eds.), *The applied theatre reader* (pp. 200–206). London: Routledge.

Hornbrook, D. (1989). *Education and dramatic art*. Oxford: Blackwell.

Jackson, A. (2005). The dialogic and the aesthetic: Some reflections on theatre as a learning medium. *Journal of Aesthetic Education, 39*(4), 104–118.

Jackson, A. (2007). *Theatre, education and the making of meanings: Art or instrument?* Manchester: Manchester University Press.

Jackson, A. (2011). Participatory forms of educational theatre. In S. Schonmann (Ed.), *Key Concepts in Theatre/Drama Education* (pp. 235–240). Sense Publishers: Rotterdam.

Johnson, L., & O'Neill, C. (Eds.). (1984). *Dorothy Heathcote: Collected writings on education and drama*. Evanston: Northwestern University Press.

McLean, J. (1996). *An aesthetic framework in drama: Issues and implications*. Brisbane: NADIE.

Neelands, J. (2011). Drama as creative learning. In J. Sefton-Green, P. Thomson, K. Jones, & L. Bresler (Eds.), *The Routledge international handbook of creative learning* (pp. 168–176). London: Routledge.

Neelands, J., & Goode, T. (2000). *Structuring drama work: A handbook of available forms in theatre and drama* (2nd ed.). Cambridge: Cambridge University Press.

O'Connor, P. (2022). Introduction to part 2. In J. O'Toole, P. Bundy, & P. O'Connor (Eds.), *Insights in applied theatre: The early days and onwards* (pp. 63–72). Bristol: Intellect.

O'Neill, C. (1995). *Drama worlds: A framework for process drama*. London: Heinemann.

O'Neill, C. (Ed.). (2015). *Dorothy Heathcote on education and drama: Essential writings*. London: Routledge.

O'Toole, J. (1976). *Theatre in education: New objectives for theatre, new techniques in education*. London: Hodder and Stoughton.

O'Toole, J. (1992). *The process of drama: Negotiating art and meaning*. London: Routledge.

O'Toole, J. (2009). Drama as pedagogy. In J. O'Toole, M. Stinson, & T. Moore (Eds.), *Drama and curriculum: A giant at the door* (pp. 97–113). Dordrecht: Springer.

Pammenter, D. (2013). Theatre as education and a resource of hope: Reflections on the devising participatory theatre. In A. Jackson & C. Vine (Eds.), *Learning through theatre: The changing face of Theatre in Education* (pp. 83–102). London: Routledge.

Pompêo-Nogueira, M. (2002). Theatre for development: An overview. *Research in Drama Education, 7*(1), 103–108.

Prentki, T. (1998). Must the show go on? The case for Theatre for Development. *Development in Practice, 8*(4), 419–429.

Prentki, T., & Preston, S. (Eds.). (2009). *The applied theatre reader*. London: Routledge.

Rasmussen, B. (2001/2022). Applied theatre and the power play: An international viewpoint. In J. O'Toole, P. Bundy, & P. O'Connor (Eds.), *Insights in applied theatre: The early days and onwards* (pp. 94–100). Bristol: Intellect.

Schechner, R. (2002). *Performance studies: An introduction* (2nd ed.). New York: Routledge.

Sinclair, C. (2006). A footprint in the mud: Entering the engaged space of community theatre practice. *NJ, the Journal of Drama Australia 30*(1), 35–46.

Slade, P. (1956). *Child drama*. London: Cassell.

Vygotsky, L. (1957/2014). *Vygotsky for education*. (Ed. Y. Karpov). Cambridge: Cambridge University Press.

Part II

The project

The wisdom of the witnesses

Part II

The project

The wisdom of the witnesses

4   What to study and who to select

Designing a training workshop

Since there is nowhere any established formal or 'objective' curriculum for applied theatre training in a community context, each facilitator has a high degree of autonomy in deciding what to teach and how. There is no 'one right way' to do applied theatre. The teaching content (what to teach) and the way of teaching (how to teach) are subjective, based on the facilitator's understanding of applied theatre and how it is learnt.

The training workshop in this study was designed to teach the general principles and practices of applied theatre, instead of – as it often is – to address a particular issue in education for development. My selection of three quite contrasting genres (*theatre of the oppressed*, *process drama*, and *participatory theatre*) to introduce in this training workshop was based on my own understanding of the potential applications in Chinese non-government organisations (NGOs) according to my previous field experience. I also intended to give the participants a variety of choices of common applied theatre strategies for their own uses.

Content and structure

The workshop was the longest applied theatre training so far in China and it took place over ten weeks, divided into three phases, each introducing one selected genre. The first and the second phase had eight sessions and the third phase had ten. Each week contained three three-and-a-half-hour sessions.

These following descriptions just identify my intentions beforehand, as the actual plan in action was allowed to be fluid and dynamic based on real-time social encounters. The detailed lesson plans were decided from week to week in consideration of the participants' responses and my increasing level of familiarity with their ability.

Phase One: theatre of the oppressed

Phase One would include theatre games and exercises, image theatre, forum theatre, and 'rainbow of desire' and 'cops-in-the-head' techniques in the training workshop. There were three dimensions to working with the group in

DOI: 10.4324/9781003426387-6

this phase: individual, group, and social. Firstly, the exercises would help to 'dynamise' the individual participants' bodies. In Boal's words, 'to be capable of making the body more expressive, first of all, control and knowledge of the body is required' (1979: 125). In addition, I hoped their growing self-understanding would help the participants begin to be aware of their strengths and weaknesses. Secondly, applied theatre is a place for collective learning. In this initial stage, the work would also serve to build the group trust and create a safe and open space for further work in solidarity. Thirdly, the central aim of theatre of the oppressed is to develop people's capacity to understand their internal and external oppression, as well as the nature of oppression in system, culture, and society. NGO workers mainly work with marginalised communities and oppressed groups. The training workshop in this phase would, I hoped, provide opportunities for them to reflect on the social situations of their clients through the activities.

Phase Two: process drama

In Phase Two, the participants would go through both the experiential and the practical stages of process drama. They would first learn from participating in several widely used 'ready-made' process dramas and then be given the challenge to plan a process drama of their own in a group. I would select dramas with diverse themes to demonstrate the possibilities of this genre. I would reflect with the participants after the experience to explore the elements of what makes a good lesson plan. I hoped the participants could gain understanding through this exploration and obtain ideas for planning their own group process drama. Then, the participant groups would try out teaching their lesson plan with the fellow participants and receive feedback afterwards.

Phase Three: participatory theatre

In Phase Three, participants would experience a collective play-making process based on those issues with which they were concerned. They would learn by doing to design activities to complement a performance involving audience participation. We would share some notions and examples of theatre for development (TfD) and community theatre at the beginning of this phase as an introduction. The role of the participants in this phase I expected to be different from the previous two phases. They would engage as teaching artists, taking various roles in the process, including playwright, actor, director, designer, facilitator, etc. They were expected to apply in preparing a performance some of the strategies learnt in previous phases, and to present that to a public audience. I did not expect them to become skilled artists; instead, through the experience of making a participatory theatre piece, I hoped to give them a sense of how applied theatre works in different ways.

My rationale for introducing those genres in that order was based on the complexities of the structure of the individual genre and how I anticipated the participants could be expected to manage it. The skills introduced in the different phases were scaffolded, rather than separately serving one particular genre. The participants started in Phase One to learn various games, exercises, and activities which were relatively easy to manage and adapt. In Phase Two, an effective process drama relies on a good framework to create a meaningful learning experience. Participants need more understanding in both applying different drama conventions and structuring the lesson plan. Content and form cannot be separated; they are mutually dependent. Learning through drama is tied to learning about dramatic form. To learn how to select and handle dramatic materials, and the skills of dramatic expression, would, I hoped, benefit participants in the third phase of their training, where outside audiences would be involved. For instance, learning the structure of forum theatre in Phase One could be applied to participatory theatre in Phase Three; learning different forms of making still images in Phase One might be a convention used to structure the Phase Two process drama experience.

Who with and where?

To ensure the workshop could be successfully organised, my choice of location was political and geographical. The study took place at Guangzhou, one of the main cities in southern China. Politically, it is the capital of Guangdong Province, which had a relatively open local policy for NGO development compared to the rest of the country at the time. There were many NGOs established and located in Guangzhou and the cities around. Local readiness was also a main reason for choosing an effective site for the research. If I chose a place where nobody knew anything about applied theatre, it would be very hard to get people to participate. In the years since Oxfam set up the first amateur applied theatre in 2005, bringing in a range of different workshops, Guangzhou has become an established foundation of applied theatre among NGOs in China. So, it was not completely new to the local NGOs. Several organisations were willing to assist the promotion of the course through their networks.

Geographically, since Guangzhou is close to Hong Kong where I live, it was convenient for me to commute between the two places; more crucially, that was important for me because under the internet censorship in mainland China it was impossible to access many websites.

Recruitment

In China, it is difficult for an individual practitioner to organise a course without back-up by a local organisation. My former partner, the Institute for Civil Society[1] of Sun Yat-sen University at Guangzhou, kindly offered to be the course's supporting organisation. Since they were one of the organisations well known for providing NGO support in China, the course information would be accessed widely, especially to reach those organisations or NGO workers unfamiliar with my name.

Course information targeting NGO workers was sent out just via email. Every applicant was required to complete a form to state their reason(s) for joining the training workshop as well as their previous drama experience, if any. I received 44 applications, including full-time NGO workers, long-term NGO volunteers, members of casual volunteer groups, tertiary students, and non-NGO people. Since the research was targeted at NGO workers, I first ruled out six applications from tertiary students and non-NGO people. Recognising the range of people working in NGOs in China, I made a preliminary short list of the rest of the applications. However, a practical training workshop could not accommodate such a large number. To make a manageable but balanced group of people from each organisation, maintaining the variety of NGOs in the training group, I finally invited 30 applicants to a briefing session, based on their expression of interest and the commitment shown in the personal statement in the application form. Prior to the briefing session, I sent a letter to every qualified applicant to clarify the foci of the training workshop. I wanted to express my intentions clearly and to invite the applicants to rethink their own. The level of commitment was a very important element to sustain the group stability of a long-term training workshop. I tried to create room for the applicants to consider their needs and establish matching expectations.

This briefing session had two objectives. First, I wanted to take the opportunity to introduce the overall structure of the training workshop in more detail, especially the purposes of the research, the participants' responsibilities, and the ethical protection for their participation. A plain language statement and a consent form were given out at the end of the session. The applicants, who were all adult professionals, made their final decision to join this three-month commitment and they all returned the consent form before they left. Second, the meeting gave the potential group members a chance to meet each other, to share their working backgrounds and express their needs and expectations for the training. It also served the purpose of warming up the participants' entry into the event. Their readiness and willingness would pave the way. It was not my intention to create a workshop merely for the research and my teaching objectives; more importantly, I was inviting them to create a space where all of us, participants and researcher alike, gained benefit from the learning process.

After the briefing session, I accepted 24 out of 30 applicants based on their level of commitment, their availability to attend all sessions, and the degree of support by their organisation, since some sessions were held on weekdays. 16 participants were full-time NGO workers working in various organisations, including three pairs and one trio of co-workers from four organisations. Three participants were long-term committed NGO volunteers and five were members of casual volunteer groups. Table 4.1 illustrates the make-up of the group and their types of work.

Two participants dropped out after the end of Phase Two due to their unexpected organisational workloads. The remaining 22 participants stayed until the end of the training workshop.[2]

Table 4.1 Participant profiles

Full time NGO workers		Long-term volunteers / casual volunteers	
# 3	org. for promoting civic society	# 4	org. for promoting rural education
# 2	org. for international poverty relief	# 2	amateur theatre groups
# 2	org. for injured workers	# 1	group for promoting environmental recycling
# 2	org. for people with intellectual disability	# 1	org. for women
# 1	org. for youth and community work		
# 1	org. for rehabilitation for mental illness		
# 1	hospital for injured workers		
# 1	org. for promoting volunteering		
# 1	org. for promoting rural education		
# 1	org for children's special education		
# 1	org. for mental health and counselling		

Source: This table identifies the parent organisations of all the Project's 24 participants.

I invited three of my Chinese students to be my teaching and research assistants in this training workshop. They helped in the tasks of video-ing and observation note-taking, as well as assisting teaching demonstrations and leading groups if necessary.

Gathering information

My training methods included: individual reflective journals, an anonymous weekly feedback form, reflection forms at the end of each phase, and a final essay at the end of the course. These were equally to assist participants' reflection, document what they had learnt, and assist me to review the teaching during the process. I collected other ancillary data during the fieldwork: my ongoing and constantly changing workshop lesson plans; visual data such as photographic documentation, drawings, objects, and images created in the workshops; artefacts produced by participants such as scripts; and their own lesson plans. My practitioner's written journal served as my own reflective record of the training workshop which I used to document my reflections on the teaching after each session, to record the participants' responses and the incidents that happened in the session. I wrote my journal simultaneously with the participants, usually scheduled at the end of a session. I also documented my reflections, thoughts, and feelings at the end of each week's interviews; informal observation notes; and video and audio recordings both of the workshop sessions and the fieldwork placements in Phase Three.

Most usefully for this book, I conducted three interviews with each participant, before, after, and again four months after the workshops, to document their chains of thought and their responses to the training workshop at different times. The first was to understand the participants' working background and their expectations and experience both in capacity building and applied theatre. The second was to understand the participants' responses to the training and their plans for applying what they had learned. The third interview was a follow-up to find out whether there was a lasting impact on the participants' learning and their use of applied theatre. After the workshop, three participants consulted me about their planning and execution of applied theatre in practice. This gave me useful insight into understanding what the participants had learned by seeing how they were already applying it.

I got a couple of unexpected bonuses in the form of longitudinal data, not planned initially, and entirely voluntary. One year after the workshop finished, I sent an email questionnaire to all participants via email. I wanted to investigate their understanding, their use of applied theatre (if any) in their own contexts, and their memories of the workshop. All 22 participants returned the questionnaires. A second bonus occurred during the writing of this book, when I attempted to contact the participants, a decade after the training. To my surprise, 14 of them responded, very willing to talk about their memories of the workshop and their own current careers. We shall share the surprising and reassuring results of these interviews in Chapter 7.

Notes

1 The Institute has now been disbanded.
2 We are going to get to know all these participants, their characters and idiosyncrasies, very well during the next three chapters, so we have given them all fictitious names.

Reference

Boal, A. (1979). *Theatre of the oppressed*. London: Pluto Press.

5 Learning applied theatre

Preamble

In this chapter, and also the next two, we are offering the reader an unusually extended acquaintanceship with the workshop participants' own words. I listened to and watched intently the development of their own capabilities and confidence through the workshop, and what they said about it and themselves. This is just a fraction of the shrewd and rapidly developing insights that I collected, which have proved to be the basis of my and my co-author's own deeper learning and reimagining of our craft. Distilling the participants' rich insights (and with their permission of course), we are sharing these with readers so that, with their own words still echoing, we can help you towards your own understanding of how to improve applied theatre practice, build practitioners' skills, and build trainees' capacity to use applied theatre effectually in whatever human service they are involved in. Throughout these chapters, we will attempt to analyse all this in a way that can provide some real-life pointers and guidelines for future applied theatre trainers and trainees.

I started with the plan to examine two overarching learning domains through the workshop: *applied theatre learning* and *generic learning*. A third, *the importance of the facilitator*, emerged spontaneously during the workshop. In the first of these chapters of 'received wisdom' we shall examine how and what the workshop participants learned about applied theatre itself.

Learning differences

In the interviews, I was intrigued by the way the beginning learners compared their learning effectiveness with those participants who had had prior applied theatre experience. This gave weight to my hypothesis that participants with differing levels of familiarity with applied theatre would be likely to be having quite different experiences, which would dictate the depth and perhaps the focus of their learning. The diversity of my volunteer group gave me ample opportunity to find out. Accordingly, I decided to divide the participants into groups dependent on their prior level of applied theatre experience. I decided on three categories:

DOI: 10.4324/9781003426387-7

- Category One – Participants with limited or no watching or participating experience;
- Category Two – Participants with a little bit of participating and practising experience;
- Category Three – Participants with participating and some practising experience.

This rough categorisation into three sub-groups served me well throughout. It did not affect my workshop planning, but allowed me to diagnose more effectively the participants' particular and differing needs, tailor the workshop accordingly and the way I dealt with the participants, and to interpret their comments accurately during and after the workshop.

The different levels of previous drama experience significantly affected the members' mode of learning, which then directly related to the depth of their applied theatre learning. I used two modes of learning: participant and facilitator. First, the *participant* mode meant that the learners mainly experienced the activities as participants and were more conscious of personal learning than thinking about applying the activities. Second, the *facilitator* mode meant that the learners experienced, observed, and analysed the activities in the process and summarised the learning in order to apply it. This kept in mind that all the participants were themselves already trainers or facilitators of some kind. These two modes of learning were not mutually exclusive, and the workshop generated both. Participant mode limits the learning mainly to superficial levels, whereas facilitator mode provides space for deeper learning how to apply theatre. All participants were to some degree using both modes. However, the dominant mode(s) of learning in each category were different.

Category One: mainly participant mode
Category Two: mixed participant and facilitator modes
Category Three: mainly facilitator mode

Category One: beginners

There were ten participants in this category, and all were beginners in applied theatre. Eight were full-time NGO workers, including three pairs of colleagues. Another two were department heads of a volunteer-based NGO (see Table 5.1 for details).

Although the Category One participants had a will to learn how to use applied theatre, they had struggles and difficulties during the learning process. Since they were new to applied theatre, most of the activities were first-time experiences for them, and they had to spend time in clarifying, so the immediate learning for them was personal. Typical was how Chenyu described himself:

When the learning process moves on, it touches my inner feeling deeper and deeper. I have been submerged in the experience and have no time to record and reflect about it.

Table 5.1 Participant profiles – Category One

Full time NGO workers	
# 2	org. for international poverty relief
# 2	org. for injured workers
# 2	org. for people with intellectual disability
# 1	org. for rehab for mental illness
# 1	hospital for injured workers
Volunteering group member	
# 2	org. for promoting rural education

Source: This table identifies the parent organisations of the Project's 10 beginner participants.

For these participants, the process was fun; they were happy and felt they were being empowered, and also challenged, in learning the new method. At the same time, they bore in mind they had come to learn how to use applied theatre. Anwen was conflicted between being a participant and learning to be a facilitator.

Sometimes I struggle and am not sure whether I am learning drama or a new working method. If I learn drama, I feel I have not much knowledge about it. I have no talent to do this since I have found myself with limited facial expression and imagination; my body is very rigid. If I learn a new working method, I don't think I am able to manage it.

Though obviously the Category One members operated in participant mode most of the time, there were a few of them placing themselves as observers during the learning process, to make sense of the methods from the facilitator's angle. There were also opportunities in Phase Two (planning and micro-teaching in process drama) and Phase Three (devising participatory theatre) to purposefully shift the members' perspectives from participants to facilitators. However, lack of previous knowledge limited their growth as facilitators, whether they intentionally observed the process or reflected after the participation. They found their understanding of the methods inadequate, and they raised a lot of questions and doubts.

The end of the session leaves many questions unresolved for me. Do I need some specific observation skills? When I was asked to make a still image, can I make whatever I want? Or should I think of a theme and make an image accordingly?

(Qiling)

Several other Category One participants expressed very similar sets of doubts and queries throughout the workshop, and the resulting feeling of inadequacy affected some of their learning confidence. Liliang and Xinhong regressed in Phase Two; and Anwen felt quite incapable in Phase Three. Jingjing found herself hardly able to make sense of the methods right from the beginning. She said she could not learn without having all the theory before the experience. In the practical exercises and placements in Phases Two and Three, the Category One members were mainly led by the experienced members in their groups.

Though there were limitations, the participants recognised the training workshop did provide them with an entry to learning about applied theatre, a change in their understanding of the basic experience and various techniques. It also gave them the chance to observe my modelling as facilitator, and some experience of the principles and pedagogy, which gave them confidence in applied theatre and motivated their continued practice.

First responses and learning the concepts

For Category One participants, their perception of 'drama' was based on the traditional view of drama as performance. As is the nature of this art form, they saw drama as a dynamic, visual, fun, expressive, attractive, creative medium. But they had no idea of the concept of applied theatre. During the learning process, they were able to gain some basic conceptual understandings about applied theatre, especially from the activities to which they felt more closely drawn.

After the first day of training, Meili had already found new applications for drama.

> *I find the applicability of drama is more than I expected to be able to use for public education. It can also help people develop empathy and has a kind of therapeutic function. I think I can use it in our new worksite and benefit the children in that area.*

and Liliang had acquired new concepts for using games:

> *I used to think games were only for ice-breaking. I had never thought of using games as strategies to help participants enter their roles.*

In the last session of Phase Two, I invited the participants to share their past and present perceptions of using drama after the two phases of training. Zhuhui and Chenyu shared their growing understanding.

> *In the past, I thought drama meant performance and only the professionals could do it. Now, I have found that drama can make things very concrete and clear, and every ordinary person can participate.*
>
> (Zhuhui)

> *In the past I thought applied theatre was a method that allowed participation. Now, I think it is more than that. Applied theatre can allow the facilitator and participants to practise for change.*
>
> (Chenyu)

Apart from the general concepts, Category One participants also revealed their learning about the concepts of the three approaches introduced.

In Phase One they tended to build their concepts according to individual exercises and activities. For example, Qiling summarised her observation on the rainbow of desire exercise:

> *The rainbow of desire is an exercise that allows the audience to try out different solutions. The protagonist can find the most suitable way to try out through watching various suggestions. We should not criticise but respect the protagonist's feeling and emotion during the process.*

In Phase Two, Jingjing wrote a good summary consolidating her learning in process drama, although she thought she had learnt very little about applied theatre.

It is important to structure a story that can engage and be understood by the participants to discuss the theme in drama.

- *The theme should be open and leave space for participants to explore different possibilities.*
- *Facilitators/leaders should hold back on expressing their own personal judgement and avoid restricting the participants' discussion. They should create an open atmosphere for the participants to explore the topics according to their interests.*
- *It is important to structure a storyline that engages participants. Conventions like defining space and teacher-in-role are strategies to assist participants to stay in role.*
- *Process drama should concern the group's common interest.*

In Phase Three, Xinhong was 'very surprised' and had a 'wonderful experience' in applied theatre after participating in and watching all three participatory theatre programs. She said the new understanding of using theatre to her was like 'turning the world upside down'.

> *In the beginning of this training workshop, I could not imagine we could create such an educational performance. My previous understanding of performance was of actors acting on stage and the audience could discuss on their own after the show. In these programs, actors could be interrupted by the audience; they could be hot-seated and say something not written on the script; and the audience could actively participate and change the protagonist's behaviour. It was unbelievable.*

Learning the techniques

It was hard for them to capture and remember all the complex procedures and patterns in their first-time encounters. Some of them could not name some strategies after the training although they had lesson plans in their hands. They were just at the stage of tasting applied theatre and at the same time learning to use it. Their lack of knowledge and experience in applied theatre made them tend to absorb the learning at surface level, i.e. the procedures and observable features of the activities. What they mentioned they had learnt were mainly the easy-to-manage single exercises, activities and conventions. One of the popular techniques was image exercises. Liliang and Zhuhui both thought about using this with their clients.

> *When I was in the 'struggling' image, I suddenly thought about my work. I could invite volunteers and clients to show factory owners and government the images of their conflicts and their relationships too.*
>
> (Liliang)

> *I can create a drama about the life of factory workers and bring it to work-ers in industrial areas. Through their interaction with the protagonists, the audience will be able to share their thoughts and solutions to the problem. It can benefit their growth.*
>
> (Zhuhui)

Although Xinhong had insufficient confidence to design a process drama, she learnt to use a simple participative storytelling technique to co-construct a story with her clients, a new experience for her. For the learning through practice, I provided the initial experience and basic knowledge for them to refer to. Anwen explained that the learning in Phase Two intro-duced her to the ideas that process drama should include a key question, scenes, roles, a framework, symbols, and drama conventions. And Chenyu learnt the structures and models of process drama from his observation of the micro-teaching.

> *I learned the importance of the step-building in process drama. The roles we set up for participants framed different kinds of possibility for exploration.*

Xinhong learnt the basic techniques of devising participatory theatre from lit-erally recalling the steps she ran through in her first experience.

> *In the last phase, we needed to collect information. Then we came back and devised our script. We reviewed the script in order to design activities to allow the audience to participate so they not only sat and watched. Therefore, we learnt how to set questions to engage and attract the audience in the process.*

Learning skills

The Category One participants learnt three kinds of skills.

Drama skills

Learning drama skills was more important to Category One participants than to the other two categories.

> *The most important learning for today was drama skills like lighting, music, rhythm and mime. It gave me a big surprise when I watched the mime presentation using the background music to create the mood. I want to use it in my future work. I want to use music to express meaning.*

> (Chenyu)

During the making process of participatory theatre, the participants mentioned they acquired some basic drama skills in devising, the uses of music, lighting and props, and stage management (e.g. scene changes and actors' entrance and exit arrangements).

Planning skills

Category One participants rarely mentioned learning planning skills. However, a few stated they gained more understanding in planning a process drama after the co-planning exercise, but they were not really able to articulate what they had learnt. Jingjing was the only one to describe her learning about planning clearly.

> *I found it was very useful to have a chance to design our own lesson plan. I learnt a lot in the process. The guiding questions in a note led my planning and it was very helpful to keep my thinking on track and not jumping around.*

Facilitation skills

Most of these participants did not consciously pay attention to my facilitation but they took notes on my methods which stimulated their thinking after the experience. In one of the image exercises, I encouraged Qiling to take risks and challenge herself to make new and unfamiliar gestures. She found my immediate encouragement to ask her to think out of the box was useful. She thought she could use this way of working with her clients to open up their minds and enhance their ability to express themselves. Minxia wanted to use the way I invited people to share ideas during group discussion.

> *I should invite every group member to take turns in sharing their feelings in my future workshops. They can use verbal or physical language. I believe it will improve their communication skill.*

After working with me to devise a short play, Zhuhui noted his learning about facilitation.

I have to consider how to help participants understand and give guidance in the devising process. I cannot impose my ideas on them. It will reduce the room for the participants to think and reflect. It will create a distance between the participants and me. If I can treat their ideas as equal to mine, they will feel accepted.

He reminded himself a good facilitator should have flexibility to adjust his plan and guidance without losing consistency.

Principles and pedagogy

In terms of learning the principles and pedagogy of applied theatre, the Category One participants were still in the process of making sense of them. Not many members clearly talked about them. Some could only generalise this area from the participant perspective. For instance, Minxia learnt about the principles from observing her own change to be more inclusive, willing to listen, respect others, be reflective; and also seeing the others' change in the process:

I learned about the principles of applied theatre from observation. I saw the change in other group members. I could also see how I practised the principles at the time I worked with others.

Zhuhui made sense of applied theatre's rationale by linking it to his organisation's work principles, after finishing the whole training workshop:

The rationale of applied theatre connects with my organisation's work principles: to care, respect and help everyone; to develop ability and potential; and to be able to solve our own problems.

Meili, who chose to pay more attention to observing teaching methods, was the only one in this category who could articulate this aspect of learning. She summarised applied theatre as participative and participant-centred. It was based on participants' active, experiential, and reflective learning. The teaching and learning relationship was equal, and all learnt together as a community through collaboration. Although the Category One participants rarely mentioned principles and pedagogy, most of them mentioned their changes in their working with clients, which I suppose was the implicit learning in the process. We will discuss this in Chapter 9.

Applying the techniques

There was limited applied theatre learning for the Category One participants, but all of them had positive comments about and trust in applied theatre after the training workshop. Some like Zhuhui felt excited by the varieties of applied theatre strategies. He described applied theatre method as a 'magic wand' which could make wonderful things.

> *I used to think the method was very rigid. I have found it to be very rich and sophisticated, but only since joining this training workshop. Previously I thought it was very simple but actually it has many layers and perspectives. This method is very deep and there is no end to the learning.*

Some found applied theatre very effective for their clients after the participatory theatre presentation in Phase Three and they generated ideas about areas where they could apply it. Minxia received positive feedback from her clients' parents after they saw their children with intellectual disabilities actively responding to the drama. She then came up with ideas where she might use drama to enhance her clients' self-care ability and social skills. Liliang gained confidence in the method, especially as there were three clients wanting to join his drama group after watching the program, which was unusual.

> *Applied theatre is not only used in promoting labour law. It has a therapeutic function. It depends on how you use it. We must fully understand our clients before we design a drama lesson plan.*

Qiling even thought applied theatre should be a prescribed skill for social workers.

> *I really think applied theatre is an effective method for my clients…drama can visualise an issue and be easy for people to receive…I believe it should be a skill for social workers. No matter whether they work with young people or like me with mental illness rehabilitants, it is a very good method. I think it will create a new page in my field if more colleagues can use it.*

Applying theatre with real people

For all participants, their level of confidence in applied theatre as an effective working method motivated their interest to practise it after the training workshop. Four factors affected their ability do so.

Job relevance

This is the first and most direct criterion for the Category One participants. Qiling, Anwen, and Minxia were required to organise workshops in their workplaces. Although they were not accomplished practitioners, they had a need to use it, and tried with their limited understanding. They used simple exercises like still image or imitating the lesson plans in the training workshop, even though they did not fully understand the principles behind them.

> *I did try to use applied theatre techniques to discuss issues with my clients.*
> *When I asked them to make a still image, they felt very uncomfortable.*
> *Because of their responses, I asked myself: 'is it suitable to use applied*
> *theatre with my clients who are mental illness rehabilitants?' or 'is only just*
> *using the still image exercise enough?' or 'is it only because I cannot man-*
> *age the techniques?'*

Apart from them, Xinhong thought applied theatre was not suitable for her clients with severe mental disability. They were not capable of articulating, expressing themselves, or managing to move their bodies very well. Her response may have come from her lack of understanding of the methods, and there was no special demonstration in the workshop on how to adjust the strategies to suit people with different abilities.

Platform

Even where there was no direct and immediate need in their regular work, some Category One participants did strive to try it out whenever there was a platform. Meili was an administrator in a youth and children's centre. She asked her colleagues to offer her a timeslot to organise a drama workshop for children during their summer holiday. Although organising social gatherings for clients was not the main job for Zhuhui, he still took the opportunity of trying out a few applied theatre exercises on one occasion. Liliang said applied theatre was not necessary to his work; however, he kept joining forum theatre performances organised by the Category Two participants. Jingjing suggested to her supervisor the inclusion of applied theatre activities in one part of the prevention training program for factory workers and managers. Chenyu thought applied theatre was irrelevant to his immediate work in an organisation and hard to use in his position; however, in his follow-up questionnaire after a year, he mentioned he was planning to include applied theatre in the new curriculum because he had thought of a place to put it in.

Availability of working partner

Job relevance was their primary driver, but some participants did need a companion. Meili was not in a position to organise workshops, although she worked in a youth and children's centre. For her colleague Anwen, who was working in the same organisation but placed in another centre, her duties enabled her to work directly with children. Anwen occasionally invited Meili to come and work with her in the centre. They discussed their plans and evaluated their attempts to implement applied theatre together. In addition, they sent me frequent emails to consult about their applied theatre work, as they thought my role as a mentor was important to support their on-going practice. Otherwise, they really didn't know how to improve their work since there was a lack of resources around their circle. Another case was Liliang, who believed in applied theatre, but he didn't think he could do it on his own. He actively joined applied theatre activities organised by others and invited other participants from the training workshop to run workshops for his clients. These kept him in touch with applied theatre practices.

The unavailability of a working partner could be a problem. Even though Xinhong and Minxia worked in the same organisation, they were in different centres and the nature of their jobs was different, which did not easily offer them the opportunity to collaborate. Furthermore, since Xinhong worked mainly with adults with severe intellectual disability, it was hard for her without any help to imagine how applied theatre might work for them without any help. Like Jingjing, she found it was 'difficult' with her limited understanding to explain the methods to her colleagues. Not being able to find a way to communicate with her working partner prevented her from practising.

Confidence

Generally, participants in this category had little confidence in using the methods because of their lack of understanding and practice as a facilitator. For some participants, like Qiling, Jingjing, Zhuhui, and Chenyu, they tried to keep practising or creating a platform for practice in order to gain more experience. The others, Meili, Anwen, Liliang, and Minxia preferred to work with each other to share their learning or invite collaboration, to assist their practice. Some of them asked for my suggestions on readings to help their own study of applied theatre.

As far as applying the methods, most of them had an awareness that applied theatre as a method is one where you use it or lose it: ongoing practice as a continued learning process was the key to enhancing their understanding. They needed to be in their own contexts to improve, since, as Zhuhui and Liliang expressed it, they found it hard to transfer exactly their learning from the training workshop into their workplaces.

> *The method is difficult to understand. It is useless if I only think about it. I should learn by doing it, discover my ability through the practice. It is the only way to learn.*

Summary: Category One

On the whole, the training workshop gave the Category One participants great confidence in the power of applied theatre. They recognised that the training workshop opened a new door of possibilities and gave them more resources for their work. At the same time, they felt it was very difficult for them to catch up with the learning:

*Too quick. I wish the workshop could be longer. For people with more expe-
rience it will be easier...it was like a running train: once the training started,
it kept running...*

(Zhuhui)

*Learning in applied theatre is like a 'bottomless hole'. Sometimes I feel
close and sometimes I feel far away from applied theatre. I have not digested
the learning yet. I am full. I cannot eat any more, but it is really very
attractive.*

(Jingjing)

They appreciated the learning and at the same time felt themselves inadequate.

*I just know of the three approaches 'at skin level'. I feel entangled and need
further learning and practice to make progress.*

(Minxia)

But most of them held the belief that applied theatre learning had had an influence on them.

*The training workshop has given me an imperceptible influence. I gained
more and more understanding about the learning as I was approaching the
end of the course. This imperceptible influence will stay deep in my heart.*

(Meili)

Category Two: a little experience

There were ten participants in this category. Five of them were full-time NGO
workers, including three from the same organisation. The other five were members of volunteer-based NGOs (see Table 5.2 for details).

Table 5.2 Participant profiles – Category Two

Full time NGO workers	
# 3	org. for promoting civic society
# 1	org. for promoting volunteering
# 1	org. for promoting rural education
Volunteering group members	
# 1	group for promoting environmental recycling
# 2	org. for promoting rural education
# 1	org. for women
# 1	Amateur theatre group

Source: This table identifies the parent organisations of the Project's 10 participants with a little drama experience.

These participants, though still beginners, had all had previous applied theatre experience. Two had some experience in theatre of the oppressed; three of them had learnt process drama before; five had experience in playback theatre and come across some drama games and exercises. Those who had less experience tended to stay longer in the participant mode, where they concentrated on their personal responses to the experience and thinking about personal issues.

First responses and learning the concepts

These participants were unlike Category One, who felt the drama activities to be alien and they were struggling to adapt. The inner struggles of Category Two members came from self-evaluation. Through their observation while participating in activities, they evaluated their own engagement and learning progress during the process. Jieyan felt good that she could be more open in the training workshop.

> *I am a slow person. I used to take 2–3 hours to open up my body. Today, I was surprised, or it was very different from before. My body was able to open up. I tried to let go [of my own desire]. In the mirror exercise, and the one-to-one activity in this afternoon, I could fully give and take…I think this workshop can help me face this issue.*

Moreover, after the end of the same session, Jieyan set herself a goal for improvement:

> *There was not much deep feeling and thinking in this session. I hope I can be in better condition tomorrow coming to the workshop. I can challenge my discomfort zone; I can have 'the third eye' to observe things and think more deeply.*

Based on their personal experience in the activities, they found benefits from the learning that drove them to apply or at least be willing to try out the activities at their workplace. Apart from their self-observation, they spent considerable time writing in the journals to record the activities. Since they came with some understanding of applied theatre, they also paid attention to my methods of facilitation.

> *How to guide through questioning? The facilitator threw the questions back to the participants. Actually, it was fully open. Let the participants think, interpret on their own. Remind them that the process of change has its own pace; we should think by stepping into other's shoes. How to do it?…The facilitator must pay attention to the meaning beyond the surface. We should create sharing time after each activity so that we can explore different points of view, learn from each other's experience, and reflect on our own views and experience.*
>
> (Yunlei)

All ten of them tried to make sense of the objectives of the individual activities by asking questions and raising queries about their uncertainties, including quite a lot of technical questions.

Oh, I had have never known there are so many layers of feeling in an event. Is the objective for using rainbow of desire and cops-in-the-head to heighten emotion? Do they want to help participants to discover and understand their own feelings? So, what is the meaning for the participants, to let them dialogue with different kinds of feeling?

(Jieyan)

I have a few questions about the rainbow of desire...does it have a therapeutic function? I felt Shuxi [the protagonist] was very brave to share yesterday. I am curious: will our clients have the same level of courage to face themselves? Or if they are willing to face themselves, can they truly articulate their feeling [in the process]? If they can't, shall I stop the story and change to another one?

(Luping)

Just after Phase One, some Category Two participants accompanied by a Category Three member initiated a study group on exploring the theatre of the oppressed. They called a meeting to collect opinions on the form, and the possibilities of sharing practices among the members. It showed the participants were beginning to take independent initiatives to search for their answers. Their prior understanding gave them a more 'trained mind'.

Learning the techniques

For these participants, there were familiar activities as well as new ones. When they revisited known activities, they did not need to remember the procedures, which spared them more time to observe and feel the activities more deeply. Yunlei said she only had superficial knowledge of Theatre of the Oppressed from her previous learning. This training workshop demonstrated to her how to dig deep on different issues by using the techniques. Now she knew how tension works in this approach and how to focus the discussion between the oppressed and the oppressor.

This was Luping's second time learning about process drama. She said that the first time she had only been able to learn what the drama conventions are and how they operate in process drama.

In this second time of learning, I learnt the importance of structuring an effective lesson plan and how we choose the focus of enquiry. A good lesson plan can engage participants to focus on a situation or a particular role's perspective; to explore the issue from different angles and different levels.

As well as learning to apply the complete approach, the participants' immediate learning included single activities and new versions of known exercises. They recorded and talked about the activities they wished to take away with them, in their journals and in discussion.

In terms of specific approaches, their learning effectiveness depended on how much opportunity they had to practise them in the training workshop. Luping and Jieyan said one demonstration was not enough to help them fully understand the techniques of theatre of the oppressed and give them confidence to try them out. However, their previous knowledge in applied theatre supported them in asking sensible questions to assist their learning.

> *What does the rainbow of desire exercise seek to achieve? What is the function of this method? How do we represent strong and weak desires? How do we transform or make a balance among them?*
>
> (Shuxi)

Shuxi had no answer for his questions yet, but obviously they were part of his learning process, kicking off his thinking and preparing him for the next experience. They acknowledged that the opportunities of practice provided in Phases Two and Three were helpful in equipping them to use the techniques.

In Phase Three, all participants learnt about participatory theatre by doing it. Four members in this category worked in one group and another two worked in another group. They were all active members in their groups. They went through the whole process of creating a program (they researched the topic, interviewed/visited the target audience, devised a play, designed interactive activities and presented the play and activities). They felt lost at the beginning but found the process of learning by doing was very helpful.

> *The process of creating a participatory theatre program was like 'pulling a bull up to the tree'. I had to do something I had never seen. Working in the unknown. Looking back, it was lucky that I did so; otherwise, I would not have such a deep understanding about this approach.*
>
> (Luping)

Starting with confusion, Luping learnt how to shape the focus of the exploration. She was chosen to be the host. At her first attempt, she did a very good job with an organised, calm, and clear mind.

Learning the skills

There were two special skills they reported they learnt in the training workshop: planning and facilitation skills. These two skills directly showed their facilitator's mode of learning.

Planning skills

The Category Two participants learnt how to create plans for their individual approaches and also learned from the overall structure of the training workshop. Luping and Jieyan specifically mentioned that they had learnt the key elements in designing a process drama. The workshop gave them many exemplars. They also learnt how to plan a drama step-by-step. Jieyan appreciated the planning and practical experience:

> *I enjoyed the process of planning and teaching. In Phase Two, I learnt: how to design a lesson plan, how to set objectives, how to reflect on our preconceived ideas and to focus the main theme. Although it was hard, I am keen to further explore this approach.*

She summarised the learning principles and applied them to her overall workshop planning.

> *It was very fundamental. It contained a lot of basic principles like setting learning objectives. That was a very stunning idea to me – starting from a question, rather than what I want the participants to do. It changes my paradigm, it is not about the message I want to give to participants; it is a co-inquiry process working together with them.*

Yunlei felt herself become more professional after the training workshop.

> *I was very messy at planning a workshop before. I had no confidence because I did not know whether I was right or wrong. Now, I know there can be many directions; the decision made depends on the context. I know more strategies and steps to assist my planning process. I feel more professional.*

Facilitation skills

All members of Category Two paid attention to my facilitation. Participants like Luping who had previous experience of some of the activities wanted to spend time on the methods of facilitation to enhance their skills. They asked questions along the way based on their experience:

> *In the making process, it is a very important skill for the facilitator to lead the group. Dealing with different kinds of topics suggested by the participants, what were the main principles and methods of facilitating the group?*
> (Xunxi)

They observed my actions and ways of responding and interacting with the group. Xunxi reflected on my facilitation and improved my flawed modelling for his own use, taking away good examples. Zhaofeng expressed fully the reason for her deep concern with the facilitation.

I chose to pay attention to what Yi-Man said, the way she said it and what she did, because this will increase my confidence as a facilitator. I can learn these skills…I want to be an applied theatre practitioner after the training workshop. I did not want just to play the role of a participant as I had in previous workshops, which did not help me to gain confidence. I wanted to observe attentively and think deeply what the facilitators did in the process, which looked like magic to me.

Learning the principles and pedagogy

This group were very attracted by the principles and pedagogy of applied theatre. All of them mentioned their appreciation and excitement in learning about it. They emphasised after the training that applied theatre is more than just a tool, it is about a set of beliefs and values to support the practice. The learning came from their first-person experience and change. From the participation, Yunlei reconstructed her experience to fit into the pedagogy of applied theatre. *The greatest learning in the workshop was gaining understanding of applied theatre pedagogy:*

- *no pre-set result; we need to create more possibilities in the process; open up thinking space for the participants and their own voice;*
- *active listening is the main skill in applied theatre; in order to effectively respond to the participants, we should have the ability to understand the feelings and thoughts behind one's speech through careful listening;*
- *observation and opening up with sensitivity are two other important skills;*
- *the facilitator should not give answers and allow rigid patterns of thought to block the learning process; more importantly, to lead the participants' reflection and ability to summarise their own learning.*

Their learning about the principles and pedagogy led to pedagogical changes in their work, which we will discuss in Chapter 9. More importantly, the confidence gained from their positive experience in the training workshop made them feel more professional in using drama.

Applied theatre allows me to see people from different perspectives. I can understand a person from his/her feelings, needs and desires. This rationale is very important in the design and facilitation of workshops. Concerns with equality, expression, personal development, reflection and how to reflect have become my work guidelines.

(Luping)

Applying theatre with real people

The Category Two participants were eager to try things out after the training workshop. Nine of the ten members in this category shared their practices with me, in interviews, questionnaire, and emails. The tenth had been busy with his leadership position, and had no time to practise. However, I received an email later that he had promoted and hosted an applied theatre workshop exploring a current matter of concern to his work.

Job relevance

These participants were independent, and they used applied theatre regardless of the nature of their job. Four members were able directly to apply the learning in their existing workplaces. They started by using the more sophisticated single games and exercises in their training work. Luping and Shuxi used physical exercises to open up the participants' bodies and minds and assisted them with self-observation. Furthermore, they used applied theatre activities whenever it suited their purpose. Shuxi and Zhaofeng found it helpful to explore social issues with young people. Jieyan used drama conventions with her participants to explore how to care for family members. Yunlei was an administrator. Although the nature of her immediate job gave her limited opportunity for practising applied theatre, she still found her own way to use it. She volunteered to lead drama activities in an organisation retreat. She actively joined colleagues from another department to use applied theatre in her spare time.

Platform

The participants in this category created their own platforms for practice. Jieyan was invited to organise for a Volunteer's Day a re-run of one of the participatory theatre programs created in the training workshop. Three members in this category joined the re-run. Shuxi, Zhaofeng and Yunlei, as colleagues, worked together in a forum theatre presentation to a group of university students. They also jointly initiated a series of applied theatre workshops in a community college run by their organisation.

Availability of working partner

Unlike the Category One participants, who required companions to motivate and assist them in applying the strategies, the members in Category Two sought working partners if there was a requirement for teamwork in approaches like forum theatre and participatory theatre. They mainly worked independently. The availability of a mentor was not an important factor in their ability to use applied theatre. Some members sent me lesson plans seeking comment and suggestions, though my presence was not a necessary factor in their decision to use applied theatre. They felt they had professional knowledge to support their practice and trusted that they would improve through ongoing practice.

Confidence

Just as for the participants in Category One, confidence was a critical factor. They expressed that they had more confidence in using applied theatre after the workshop, although they did not fully understand every method.

> *The training workshop brought me great motivation to practise. I want to use the strategies I learnt in the workshop. I am more ambitious and have more confidence to try out applied theatre. Though I can only use the forms and sometimes I am not sure of the functions of the activities, I am still keen to use applied theatre when I want to stimulate participants' thinking and make change.*

> (Jieyan)

Jieyan did not have confidence in all the activities taught in the workshop. She expected she would gain more courage to try out other methods after accumulating more experience, and she believed that practice was the golden key to internalising applied theatre. Although she mentioned failure in her practice work, she did not give up using it. Similarly, Luping had an unsuccessful experience in practice, but the professional knowledge she had gained in the workshop gave her confidence to improve the next time.

Successful practice, certainly, is a good way to bring confidence. Yunlei used image exercises in her organisation retreat. She obviously felt she was now different and readier to lead the exercises.

> *I felt so good. I did not feel shy or nervous. It was so smooth. I know how to give instructions, compared to the past, where we would ask someone who was more experienced to lead the activities. But now, I am confident to do it by myself.*

No matter whether their practices failed or succeeded, it seemed that the confidence gained from the training workshop made them trust applied theatre, which created a force to move them forward to be willing to take risks and try out new strategies. Zhaofeng, for example, was so excited about applied theatre that she felt she could use everything learnt in the training workshop.

> *Applied theatre really works. My belief is based on my personal understanding, connection and change in the process. And also it comes from seeing other people's change in the workshop. I am so confident and think I can design and facilitate applied theatre workshops.*

Her high personal confidence was reflected in her practice and her progress. She used image exercises just after the training workshop and was not very successful. Then she used drama in a sharing event with partners from other organisations and received much positive feedback. With increasing confidence, she used image exercises again and this time she found her skill more mature. From applying single exercises, she tried to conduct and design her own process drama workshop. The ongoing practice played an important role in her professional development.

Summary: Category Two

The techniques, skills, rationale, and pedagogy that the Category Two participants learnt from the training workshop, on top of their previous learning, brought them to another level of understanding applied theatre. They told me they had used the methods superficially in the past. They blindly imitated what they had seen and experienced in previous workshops without knowing the rationale and pedagogy behind the strategies; one had even thought applied theatre activities were just for fun. After the training they found they had more ideas and a clearer rationale to support their practice.

> *In my past learning in applied theatre, I could only imitate. Now I want to explore more. I really want to use this method. I will ask myself, 'why do I want to use some specific strategy?' I wouldn't ask this question before, but I am now more accomplished. After learning from experience, I know how to react in an emerging situation and give a prompt response.*
>
> (Shuxi)

Most importantly, they could feel a sense of professional growth.

> *In these ten weeks of training, I became in touch with applied theatre and got to know its theory. I had opportunities to practise, and it increased my understanding of how to apply it. I have more confidence. Although my skill is still immature and raw, I know which the right direction is.*

The growth also came from questions, confusions, and unknowns. Jieyan mentioned that the more she explored applied theatre in depth, the more questions were raised in her mind. She affirmed that this process had the capacity to broaden her vision.

> *I cannot use all the techniques at the moment. However, the learning process kept stimulating my thinking. It gave me different ways to observe applied theatre. This thinking process is very crucial. Now I know we have to make professional decisions to choose what to use. I gained more understanding after our exploration. It has opened my vision.*

Zhaofeng asked the question of how to integrate the principles into the activities, which was very fundamental to her further professional development.

I now know the principles, but I think I still need time to further explore their application.

Though participants were not able to become accomplished in all methods, they tended to make more informed choices in using the strategies, selecting those activities more in line with their own ability, understanding, needs, and contexts. Their professional confidence increased. They used the methods with more understanding, and the assurance of ongoing practice as a way of learning applied theatre.

Category Three: more experience

There were two members in Category Three, Baiyi and Tianxin. They had experience of attending different kinds of applied theatre and facilitating workshops. One was a full-time NGO worker in a social organisation and the other one a volunteer, an active member of an amateur theatre group and herself a staff member in a commercial company (see Table 5.3 for details).

Both arrived with many questions. They mentioned in the first interview that they would like to have more systematic learning in applied theatre. They had been learning about applied theatre through attending and facilitating workshops, as well as participating in interactive theatre for a number of years. They felt unsatisfied and dried-out in practice, which drove them to come to this workshop for further development in applied theatre.

From the beginning of the workshop, they were in facilitator mode. Apart from their eagerness to learn more new activities, they also set their own learning focuses in the process. Baiyi concentrated on understanding the principles of applied theatre and the facilitation skills. Tianxin's emphasis was on building her own theory of applied theatre. Therefore, what they learnt from the training workshop, which blended the concepts, techniques, skills, principles, and pedagogy, did address their focus, in the main.

Baiyi had attended workshops about theatre of the oppressed before. He placed his main attention on the methods of facilitation and the structure of the lessons right from Phase One.

Table 5.3 Participant profiles – Category Three

Full time NGO workers	
# 1	org. for youth and community work
Volunteering group member	
# 1	amateur theatre group

Source: This table identifies the parent organisations of the Project's 2 participants experienced in applied theatre.

How can we run an effective workshop with participants from a range of backgrounds? When we play games in the workshop, how can we experience and accept cultural respect and understanding?...

...Will we create memories of the process of having physical connection with others that influence our thought?...

...What is the right time to give suggestions? How can we catch the main points for the exploration of issues from the participants' conversations?

Apart from that, he also mentioned his self-observation during the process and linked it to his professional development.

To be true to self and take the risk of expressing oneself...Expression is a process to promote relationships. It can help to strengthen the theatre skills and create a sense of security for the participants.

Tianxin did not have as much experience in the theatre of the oppressed as Baiyi. She knew some games and image exercises from previous courses and had once done a forum theatre presentation within a workshop. She described them as glimpses of the approach. Therefore, this phase of learning for her comprised a mix of familiar exercises and completely new activities. She chose to reflect on the meaning of activities. She was focused on making sense of every activity and she tried to articulate their objectives afterwards. She puzzled over those activities with complex structures. She was unsure how to make the rainbow of desire exercise work after watching it only once. During the small-group work, she felt it was hard to devise an effective scene to provoke discussion and intervention for forum theatre.

Like Baiyi, she raised the question of how to facilitate:

If we work with beginners, should we first help them to open up their body, to stimulate them by using games? Then we can ask them to create still images and sculptures, to imitate, share and express by using their bodies? And what about other drama work afterwards? How can I guide this process? What is the most effective way to facilitate participants?

It was she who joined some of the Category Two members in organising a self-study group for theatre of the oppressed. She was also invited to share her own practice and she led a session on using image exercises for the group members. She took the initiative for her own and others' learning.

Process drama was new to Baiyi. Like other participants, he commented on his acting limitations, and he shared their mixed feelings about role in the experiential period.

It was hard to jump into a role in a short time. I think it may be lack of experience in life.

He was not very active in this phase, as he himself admitted:

I was absent for some sessions in this phase. I felt behind.

From his limited participation, observation and listening to others in discussion, however, he got a basic grasp:

Process drama places the participants at the centre. It allows participants to feel the characters in role. It is easy to engage in the drama…

In contrast, Tianxin was excited by process drama. She was not new to it, and she built on her previous learning. Right from the beginning. she put her focus on the structure of lesson plans and facilitation.

I paid great attention to how the facilitator structured the drama and linked up different parts…
Using the materials from real life in drama was very effective. It provides a thinking space for participants. It will touch and affect people.

She found the planning and practical period was very helpful.

I made painstaking efforts to finish the design of the lesson plan for micro-teaching. It was an important process for learning. No matter whether you decide to use a convention or not, it is all the matter of linking with the teaching objective.

And she gained more confidence in using process drama.

I feel happy. The opportunities to experience many different lesson plans broadened my mind. I feel more solid…I have more confidence to design my own plan…
I like the process of learning (experience, planning, and practice). I want to use the lesson plan designed by my group later, with outside participants.

Both members of Category Three had previous experience in play-making and participating in interactive theatre performance. They naturally took active leading roles in their groups, especially in helping to direct the drama. Baiyi worked in the group creating a participatory theatre piece targeted towards adults with intellectual disability. He thought he understood the participants very well since he had worked with similar kind of clients before. However, it was not the case in practice. He realised that he was used to working with 'talented' clients who were highly selected.

In Phase Three, my knowledge about the clients was very superficial. Actually, I may only have known 5% of them, which I used to think was already very representative.

He then wrote about new understanding about working with clients that he had gained from the practice:

> *I need to learn to be more attentive, more focused; to see things from stepping into others' shoes, from the perspective of my clients.*

He also mentioned self-observation in the process as well as working in a team.

> *I discovered some of my characteristics in the process. I sometimes lost my temper, sometimes I was too casual and reserved. In the beginning I thought it would not be too hard since I had previous experience. Actually, it is always different when you work with a new team. Anyway, I felt very satisfied with the performance. We all performed very well according to what we had to offer. I did a lot of reflection and I improved.*

At the beginning, Tianxin shared responsibility with her group members. However, the members (most of them Category One participants) were confused by the key objectives of the program. They did not clearly understand the issue being presented to the audience. Tianxin took up the leading role when the group got stuck. Mid-way through she asked me for a meeting to consult how she could do this, in which she organised her ideas and suggested a work plan to send to all members. She came back the next week and improved the working efficiency of the group.

> *Overall, it was good although the process was not so smooth. We made many mistakes. One statement by Yi-man has had a great influence on me, 'Have you placed your clients into your heart?' In other words: Do we see them as a concept or a group of people we serve? I found our mistakes also related to this. We did not put them at the centre of our program design. It will affect my way of doing participatory theatre in future.*

In general, the learning of the two members in this category built on their previous experience. Besides personal learning from the experience, they obviously reflected and commented on the activities from a facilitator's point of view. They spent time observing my methods of facilitation and were conscious not to over-talk during group discussion. They were relatively more able to make sense of the learning on their own. As Tianxin wrote on the first day of the training workshop:

> *We need to experience, reflect, summarise, and consolidate the learning in order to construct our learning through the integration of experience and theory. Carrying our own theory, we can understand how to apply different approaches and games into our practice.*

They asked themselves questions about the skills and techniques of application, although they may not have found answers. Although they were not fully expert in every strategy, especially for those methods they were encountering for the first time, their responses were different from the other two categories. They did not feel frustrated nor lose their learning confidence like the Category One participants. They did not actively ask technical questions to clarify the procedures and details of the approaches like the Category Two participants. The Category Three members tended to contemplate in internal reflection, or simply make their own choice about what they wanted to further develop. This may explain why they mentioned learning as a facilitator and about applied theatre as an ongoing business.

> *I want to discover and nurture myself to be more careful about details, to be attentive; to carry a sense of equality and harmony without losing humour. The key to achieve it can only be based on the facilitator's personality. It is the process of gradual development. This is a lifetime assignment. Never-ending. The more I learn about applied theatre, the less I know. I feel myself rather like a beginner, and I never finish learning.*

(Baiyi)

Summary: Category Three Participants

Baiyi

Baiyi chose to 'hold two minds' in the learning process. One mind was for observing himself in action; the other mind was for observing others (participants and facilitator). He emphasised his improvement in active listening skills.

> *In this 10-week workshop, I gradually gained the ability to understand the meaning beyond one's speech. I can tell better why someone says what they say and understand that in terms of their belief and background.*

He also applied this skill in the workshop to actively listen to what I said, and he made the following comment about being a facilitator.

> *Being a facilitator, we need to observe ourselves. We should know why we choose to say something or not; why we speak this instead of that; what is the reason behind it; how we choose to respond or not respond to the participants.*

In the questionnaire one year after the workshop, he noted that he treasured this active listening skill. He also said, 'Actively listening to what other people say has become my habit'.

The workshop provided Baiyi with a space for observation. Like a witness, he could see the organisation of the workshop as well as the learning of other members. He was able to assess the participants' learning from observing their bodies' flexibility. He mentioned 'I learned how to set up activities and these details of facilitation can help me to understand how to open up the participants' ability.'

Apart from the facilitation skill, his experience of practising participatory theatre gave Baiyi a different angle to see how to work with clients. He found he had only known his clients superficially before this practice. He learned the importance of client-centred planning which focuses on the needs of participants. This idea replaced his original facilitator-centred planning, and deepened his future practice.

Regarding the learning of applied theatre strategies, he recorded bits and pieces of new games and exercises in his journal for future reference. He mentioned that the training workshop refined and deepened his existing knowledge, especially of how to devise an open and effective forum theatre. Process drama was new to him, and he had missed a few sessions. He did not feel confident enough to develop a lesson plan. However, unlike the beginners, he showed the ability to build on a surprising understanding of process drama – given his absences.

> *Through the detailed set-up and teacher-in-role in process drama, participants can deeply explore their inner feelings, which stimulates further discussion and generates new possibilities and new understanding. The facilitator starts with using one or more pre-texts, allowing the participants to experience different roles in the process (create empathy), letting them see a problem from different angles...*

He was an experienced practitioner and received frequent invitations to conduct workshops. So, he got many opportunities after our workshop to use applied theatre as part of his job. In his report, he did not indicate that he had used any specific approach from the workshop. He took the activities learnt from the workshop as his reference points and used whichever of them were suitable to his own workshop's objectives and contexts. However, the facilitator qualities he developed through his observation and reflection continued to contribute to his work. He said in the questionnaire after a year:

> *The training workshop gave me confidence. I can be more attentive to understand how the participants think and feel. I have self-confidence that my workshop can bring benefit to others.*

This new confidence was one of the catalysts that drove him to become a full-time freelancer one year after the training. He also actively sought opportunities to do further study in applied arts overseas.

Tianxin

Tianxin gave her attention to the activities and the principles behind them. She was keen to build her own sense of the different approaches. As she said:

> *I only learnt about the forms and methods without understanding their principles before. In this training workshop, I was able to learn about the framework of applied theatre as well as its rationale, which enhanced my professional ability.*

She acquired deeper understanding of the techniques she had already known, like still image and process drama. She had previously utilised still image as an activity to kill time in the workshop. Whenever she did not know what to do, she would ask participants to create an image. But now, after she had experienced the variety of uses of still-image exercises within the workshop, she realised it was an effective strategy to connect and communicate with people. Furthermore, she had a breakthrough in learning process drama, of which her previous workshops had left her with only blurred understanding. In this workshop, the experience itself, and her micro-teaching opportunity, built on her existing knowledge.

> *I think the second phase brought me fun and broad experience of process drama. I participated in many lesson plans; and then I tried out planning and teaching which gave me confidence. I have learnt how to select pre-text and practice better. I like this form very much. I want to use the plan we designed with 'real' participants.*

She also actively built up her understanding of new strategies. She was very engaged in the learning process. Besides taking copious notes of the new games and exercises, she recorded questions and reminders for future practice in the journal after every experience. She summarised her learning as a record of 'this stage of the process' so that it could provide a basis for the next time. She did not just learn how to operate activities, but at the same time she was constructing for herself an overall concept of applied theatre.

> *Applied theatre is not like the traditional teaching method. It sets up scenes for discussion and sharing. Participants think and learn from experience. Applied theatre provides a safe space to help them to face and solve problems.*

Like Baiyi, she too was attracted by the client-centred planning approach, especially after the Phase Three practice.

> *Yi-man asked me, 'Do you put the clients into your heart?' This statement had a great impact on me. Do I treat the clients as an object or a subject? This does matter. I find myself making mistakes every time because I do not put my clients at the centre of planning'.*

These concepts and planning principles were to lead to changes in her practice.
    Tianxin gained great satisfaction from this training workshop. Her enhanced knowledge about applied theatre and the changes which she had noticed in

other members in the process gave her confidence in her own ability to apply it. This confidence drove her, after the workshop, to resign her job in a commercial firm and become a full-time applied theatre practitioner. Working as a full-time practitioner, she had many opportunities to put her new knowledge into practice. She actively applied her learning from the workshop, especially process drama. She was practising this form by using others' lesson plans, and also creating her own plans.

Through the practice she felt more able to manage the form. Later, she also participated as one of the leading organisers in re-running a participatory theatre program originally created in the training workshop. In the rehearsal process for that re-run, she told me she suddenly realised 'all three phases of learning in the training workshop actually linked with each other'. She utilised the games and exercises more flexibly and better integrated for her purposes, except 'rainbow of desire' and 'cops-in-the-head', which she thought she needed still more time to make sense of.

Baiyi and Tianxin both showed their learning process was more self-directed, based on their background, interest, and experience. They both emphasised that the more they learned, the more inadequate they felt their own professional skills were.

Applied theatre is very beautiful. It works! Applied theatre is so big and it attracts me to move forward. I am so small and need more learning. Applied theatre gives me confidence for further development.

(Tianxin)

Learning about applied theatre is 'a lifetime assignment'. This ability can only be gained from participating in and facilitating workshops. You can never learn just from your imagination; it won't help you improve.

(Baiyi)

These frank, self-critical, and revealing comments achieved what I had wanted most from the workshop: to provide a basis for understanding not only how and how much people learn in applied theatre, but also how the participants increased their own capacities and how much might be sustainable in their futures.

6   Generic learning

Preamble

Just as the professional learning in applied theatre that we discussed in the previous chapter distinctly showed up the differences in the three categories of participant, I was able to identify that there were three distinct kinds of generic learning for the participants which were not nearly so dependent upon their previous level of applied theatre experience. These are:

- Personal learning,
- Pedagogical learning, and
- Reflective learning.

The participants described that they had not expected to encounter these kinds of learning before they came to the training workshop. Although they clearly identified these three generic learning types in their interviews as well as in the final essay, they could not articulate all the specific moments or activities when this learning was taking place. This profoundly reflects the tacit nature of the generic learning embedded in the training workshop. Some participants were specifically influenced by one category of generic learning and made little or no mention of the other kinds. Nevertheless, it is still important to start from their perspectives: recording in this book how they accounted for their generic learning, and the ways they described how the learning changed their understanding, attitudes and behaviour, both at work and in life, provides critical clues to deepening our own understanding of the whole learning process.

Personal learning

All participants mentioned that they gained some personal learning in the training workshop. A representative comment made by Minxia described her impression of the personal learning impact on the group:

> *I don't think we were in a training group. Instead, we were a personal development group. Because every time I came, I found people changed.*

DOI: 10.4324/9781003426387-8

However, because of the tacit quality of the learning, only a few of them were able to document what influenced their personal learning in the training process. So, their responses mix in descriptions of what they learnt and how they felt in the training workshop, as well as their changes at work afterwards. They most often mentioned these main types of personal learning.

Self-awareness

> *The whole training workshop made me form a habit of seeing and observing myself.*

This comment from Shuxi was common to most of the participants. They felt impressed by the opportunities to enhance their self-awareness, and that allowed them to observe and understand their inner feelings, and to know more about their own limitations and habitual behaviour.

Recognising inner feelings

The participants felt touched by the experience enough to dig deep into their own inner feelings. As Anwen said, she started to become aware of her feelings and to think about them during and after the workshop. She gained self-understanding from this awareness.

> *I was able to discover some things that have existed in my heart for a long time. I did not know they have been living with me for so long. Didn't have a chance before to see how I was blocked – to find out the reason why I have grown like this.*

Qiling told me she had always neglected her feelings before. She seldom dared to express them and used to suppress them. She learnt from the discussion sessions and the drama activities that she should value her own needs and feelings. She started trying to admit and deal with her feelings, positive and negative. She found benefits from this change:

> *If I can be more concerned about my personal feeling, I can find the clue to what makes me feel uncomfortable and then I can take care of myself. If I can observe my emotion, I can discover more about myself and promptly find a way to deal with it.*

Importantly, she found this capacity contributed to her work. She found she was able to be more sensitive and empathise with her clients when they shared their puzzlement and what made them unhappy. Zhaofeng extended this idea to link the importance of self-awareness to the basic qualities for NGO/social workers.

I found it was a fundamental experience in the training workshop to discover oneself…I think this is so important to everybody who works as NGO or social workers, and it is always missing in our field. From caring and understanding ourselves, we can understand others.

Knowing one's habitual behaviour and limitations

Apart from feelings, the participants discovered their limitations and their behavioural patterns when they interacted with others. Through self-observation, they had opportunities to re-learn about themselves. It was an important element to enable change. Chenyu found that habitually his mind kept tight control over his body during the exercises. Although he could not liberate his body in this short time, he recognised that applied theatre would help him to achieve this goal.

I think I will be able to liberate my body eventually. The training workshop helped me to understand myself. To understand what has been controlling me was the starting point to think how to release these locks. And I know applied theatre can be a safe place for me to learn how to liberate myself. I may not do it in real life, but I am sure I can do it on stage.

A great impact on Baiyi was his new understanding of his expressive ability. He originally thought he was good at expressing himself. During his own observation in the training workshop, he was surprised he was not as capable as he had thought. This new understanding created a drive to improve.

Because I know my real level of ability, I can use it seriously to improve. Had I kept thinking I was good enough, I wouldn't have made any improvement.

Unlike Baiyi, Jieyan found she had a habitual mode of thinking that only focused on seeing negative things, which made her always feel frustrated. With this observation in mind, she reminded herself not to neglect the positive side, and to keep balanced perspectives. Zhuhui too recognised that he tended to hold negative emotions and ignore the clients' feelings during their discussions. The training workshop enhanced his sensitivity to observe his own emotional cycle so that he could manage his negative emotions and change his relationship with his clients. He described it was a process of 'cleaning'.

It touched my heart. I felt refreshed. As if old dust has been cleared. I feel as if I have been promoted after cleaning out that old and accumulated rubbish.

Knowing their habitual behaviour also impelled the participants to try out new responses in the training workshop. Shuxi observed he always feared to be seen and exposed doing exercises in public. He found there were lots of inner mind controls blocking him and keeping him distanced from others. He resisted others' ideas. Although he did not expect to be able to make a sudden change, the intensive opportunities in the workshop to observe himself were very meaningful for him. The realisation was a critical prerequisite for him to make decisions. He did attempt to open up himself in the training workshop.

> *I found a change. I used to resist different opinions. I always held on to my idea tightly…In Phase Three, I was very resistant in the discussion where we chose the topic for our participatory theatre program. I recognised my resistance. In the past, I would persuade others to accept my idea. This time, I gave way to others' ideas and opened myself up to try them.*

Self-confidence

The participants described their increasing self-confidence during the training workshop. They found they were more willing to express themselves publicly, be more assertive, and feel able to change. From the participants' revealing responses, there were three kinds of forces contributing to improving their self-confidence.

First, some mentioned that it was important to see others being brave in the learning process and in their practice. They appreciated other members – including me as facilitator – being willing to take risks, and they took it as a cue to act differently. Before the first activity started in session one, Xinhong challenged me about wasting so much time in checking the expectations of the group. Some participants wrote in their journal, praising her braveness in challenging the teacher, which was unusual in Chinese culture. After the rainbow of desire exercise in Phase One, many participants admired Shuxi as the protagonist who disclosed his sexual orientation. On another day Shuxi also shared his innovative social projects with the others. Jingjing was impressed by his courage, and that affected her own change:

> *When I get back to my workplace, I can be more assertive. I am braver in expressing my opinion. I think this courage comes from Shuxi's work, especially how he responded to social issues in action. I was moved by him. So, when I get back to work…when I see something unfair, I will stand up and fight to counter it now.*

During the encounters with others, Chenyu felt deeply he had ability to make change in himself.

> *I had thought I quite understood myself. I was honest in facing my problems. However, I was missing the ability and the way to make changes. After this training workshop, I feel I am able to make changes. It was because I saw the courage of others, and through them I saw myself. I learnt about myself through other people's stories. The experience gave me more strength.*

Second, the culture within the training workshop of encouraging expression also played a role in enhancing participants' self-confidence. Meili, Anwen, and Qiling mentioned that they had obviously changed to be more willing to express their viewpoints publicly. Qiling compared this with her responses in the past:

> *I would not expose myself, because I was afraid I might be wrong. I was not certain about my ideas. Now, I find I feel more comfortable to speak out and actually my opinion is workable.*

Third, the opportunities in the training workshop to practise helped the participants to create self-confidence. Yunlei found the opportunities for acting and presenting made her more active and confident. She explained in detail how the gain in confidence changed her way of work.

> *Acting and presenting boosted my confidence. I was a passive person and did not dare to stand out to show my ability. Although I am a person-in-charge of an administrative department, I always retreated. I preferred to invite people from outside to take up my training jobs. When I decided on a course, I usually preferred to be a coordinator not the facilitator. After this training workshop, I think I can try to stand in the front.*

Six months after the training workshop, she confirmed the change in herself:

> *I became more mature after the training workshop. Learning from lots of dialogues and open sharing, I found my work style gradually changed...I have gained more confidence. I can have more sense of control at work and feel work is smoother and more effective.*

Social ability

The training workshop incorporated many different kinds of interactive activity, which the participants identified as enhancing their social ability to express themselves, to listen, and to care for and empathise with others. They also talked about this type of personal learning based on sharing their attitudinal and behavioural changes at work.

To express

Participants valued applied theatre training as it was able to enrich their ways of expression, not limited to verbal language. Luping brought up this point clearly:

> *I only relied on verbal language before. This training workshop made me see how important it is to use physical language. It can provide me with an additional way of expression.*

Chenyu, a participant who much appreciated the artistic ways of expression, described how learning new ways to express himself would contribute to his life.

Influenced by my past education, I found using verbal or written language were not enough to express myself, especially my feelings. So, I had strong expectations that I was going to learn an art form that would help me to express myself. Through rich expression, I can be relaxed, re-experience, promote and liberate myself…the different kinds of physical exercises in the training workshop made me feel very nervous because I had forgotten how to use my body, how to control my body to complete tasks. Therefore, I am very sure this is what I needed to learn.

To listen

In the training workshop, by the nature of applied theatre pedagogy and the way I structured their work, the participants had to work collaboratively with each other in different formats such as pair work, small-group planning, whole-group sharing, and discussion. During this process, they were given opportunities to learn how to listen to others and respect others' opinions. As Meili said,

The collaborative opportunities in the training workshop made me slow down and listen to others attentively. I found everyone was very smart. Creating things with others always achieved better work than merely working on my own. I am more willing to listen and accept others' ideas.

Anwen described how she changed her attitude to working with others.

When I discussed with people in the past, I found it easy to be impatient. I only wanted others to listen to me and accept my ideas. Now, I am not like this. No matter whether I am in the training workshop or back in my workplace, I can be patient in sharing my views…let other people finish their point and I can try to think about their stance…

By making similar changes at her workplace, Minxia described her colleagues' responses to those:

My colleagues felt my change, change to be more gentle. They said I used to be a dominant person and impose my ideas on other people. Now, they have found I will share my views and experience, and at the same time allow others to express their views.

To empathise

Most of the participants found they could be more caring and empathic towards other people after the workshop. They could think from another's perspective – not just hold tight to their own views, but respect others' needs and give others space (Anwen, Xinhong, and Xunxi were among those who explicitly commented on this). These changes generated a positive impact for their personal relationships. Meili explained that through an interaction in role she could regain the feeling of a heartfelt encounter. It inspired her to work with clients differently in future. Chenyu further explained that the practice in the training workshop helped him to understand the core value of working with people.

I have gained more understanding about people. I remember the word 'magic' [the specialised term from theatre of the oppressed to label inauthentic action]. It reminds me it is impossible to expect people to do what we want. We should understand others' pain. To empathise is the core value of our work…this training workshop gave me concrete and deep experience to learn about it…I learnt how to care for others in my organisation…

Zhuhui even mentioned his behavioural change at work.

If my clients distrusted and resisted our help in the past, I would simply think this was their problem. I would criticise them. But now, I will consider that they may be rejecting me because – like the stories in our dramas – they may have had something that happened before which causes their distress. They need my help.

He was also surprised by his change to naturally sit closer to his clients, whereas before he only stood at the door of the ward talking to his clients in hospital.

Now I want to sit closer to them. I did not have this feeling before. I think if we can shorten the distance between me and them, I can feel their needs, 'read' their feelings and get more understanding about them.

Pedagogical learning

This generic learning has already been mentioned in the last chapter. Reviewing the participants' responses, I found that learning the principles and pedagogy of applied theatre was common to all participants, in all categories. Although the contents of the pedagogical learning the participants mentioned, such as democratic, dialogic, reflective, experiential, and people-centred learning, are similar, the application discussed in this section is slightly different. Here, I am referring to the wider scope of application through which the participants learned to use the pedagogy in general and not necessarily just as it relates to applied theatre. Obviously, the Category Two and Three participants made more explicit mention of this kind of generic learning. They could also refer to the positive learning they had gained from previous applied theatre experience. They had some sense of the pedagogical principles of applied theatre, which they appreciated, and they put the focus on those.

To a certain extent, the Category One participants were attracted by applied theatre pedagogy before they came to this training workshop. Although not every member in this category could articulate their pedagogical learning, it affected them all at a different level. Three out of ten did emphasise their pedagogical learning and described how it impacted on their practice. Another five did not specially mention it, but it was implicitly shown from the examples they gave about new ways of practice, such as involving collaboration and participation, and client-centred planning. Two participants who found difficulties in learning applied theatre did not think they had gained any pedagogical learning. However, from how they described their own learning experience, I can see they did gain some benefits, like teaching more effectively through visualisation and learning from others. They lacked the ability to integrate their personal positive experience into their understanding of how they were applying it.

Overall, the participants claimed their own pedagogical learning came through personal experience and observation of other participants' changes during the workshop; and also the change following the workshop in their own way of thinking and practice at work.

I was next able to identify six aspects of pedagogical learning and how the participants accounted for the influence of these on their practice.

Change in understanding of pedagogy

Participation and empowerment

Participants described that the embodied experience of participation and empowerment in the training workshop changed their way of working, whereas before, they had only had intellectual understanding of these concepts.

> In order to empower the clients, we should let go of our egos as facilitators. I had learnt this concept intellectually in the past. After the experience in action, I found it is not as easy as I thought to really give the power back to the clients. Beforehand, I was the one in a group who gave lots of suggestions; now, I will give more space for the clients' suggestions and together we can try them out.
>
> (Qiling)

Like Meili, Qiling changed her way of leading the drama group at her centre. She used to set a fixed script for the group members to follow but from now on she would co-devise the play with them. She found this increasing degree of participation made the members more engaged in the process. It satisfied her to watch them shift from being uninterested to active participation. Zhuhui further articulated the importance of involving participants in the teaching process, based on his learning in the workshop.

*The workshop made me think more deeply about working with clients.
I think of how I can help them to understand things or guide them in a new
direction. I should not ignore their ideas and their process of reflection by
imposing my ideas or giving them answers. To do this will create a distance
between me and them. If we can have a more equal relationship, the clients
will accept each other with a good grace.*

Engaging the participants can also happen in the process of teaching. Jieyan
was attracted by setting questions instead of statements as her teaching objectives. This was a completely new idea for her.

*Starting from questions means the learning does not have to be based on
what I want to do with the participants. To change my way of thinking:
learning is not about sending my message to the participants, it is an
exploration, working together with them...this leads me to think of the
position of the participants and of me as facilitator in the process.*

People-based pedagogy

Participants mentioned that applied theatre gave them a platform to focus,
explore, and empathise with people's feelings, needs, and desires. It was not an
idea or an attitude that emerged through talk or seminar; this learning was
manifested in action. It triggered them to think from their clients' perspectives.

*Applied theatre gave me many ideas, especially how to understand people.
I find it's very useful; it is valuable to understand people's feelings, needs
and desires. Because I am a social service worker, this learning can help me
design my workshop better.*

(Luping)

*To see people's need is an important starting point, especially for my work.
Before, I had only learnt from theory but now I can learn from my own
experience. It is very fundamental to how to understand people.*

(Zhaofeng)

Learning to understand others' feelings helped the participants become more
considerate to their clients. They learnt to respect their individual differences,
personalities and personal habits. Instead of setting all teaching objectives
based on the facilitator's agenda, they now started thinking from the participants' point of view. Meili shared her pedagogical change:

*Now, I design activities based on my participants' desires and needs. I pre-
viously thought they came to my workshop only for the gifts. Now I think
about it from their situations. I wonder what they would want after a long,*

tiring day's work. How can I engage them? I am more active in trying out different ways to communicate with them. I have changed from merely being concerned about their materialistic needs, to their spiritual needs.

Culture of learning

Some participants appreciated and enjoyed the culture of learning. They described how the training workshop made them learn the essence of applied theatre, which is dialogical, respectful, equal, and open. They learnt by living through the process. As Zhaofeng said,

> *I experienced what equality was about in the process. Equality doesn't mean that everyone gets the same thing. It means we can pay respect to every member's experience and also their past. We can all choose what we want to see, feel and learn.*

Luping mentioned that the philosophy she learnt in the workshop affected her way of thinking at work. She said,

> *I apply the essential principles more consciously, like emphasising reflection, equality and dialogue, giving everyone a space to develop, listening actively when I am planning or conducting a meeting.*

Collaborative learning

Participants felt impressed by the many opportunities for collaboration throughout. They frequently worked with people in different forms of collaboration like pairs, small groups, and the whole group. They found the collaborative setting helped them to learn how to express themselves and listen, as well as to learn from others' ideas. They discovered they were learning not only from me as the facilitator, but from everybody in the group.

> *I found every member in this training workshop was very distinctive. Unlike the previous workshop I attended, this time I found we built the knowledge together. Everybody was a treasury and shared their 'precious stones' with each other. Very rich! I learnt not only from the facilitator. I saw everybody had some contribution to make, to produce the knowledge. It greatly inspired me – the facilitator of a workshop does not own it; more importantly, s/he must stimulate the participants to work together. The result will be much richer.*
>
> (Luping)

Self-constructive learning

Some participants described that the 'self-constructive' method of learning in the training respected every learner's pace, which created more learning possibilities for them. Meili reflected:

The learning content was not like the textbook which is restricted by its fixed script. The learning progressed through individually documenting our feelings and thoughts in the reflective journal; then sharing, summarising and consolidating the learning through group discussion, which was able to help to ease my doubts and remove blind spots in my own private thinking. No standard answer was provided; the learning was full of possibilities.

For Zhaofeng, this learning process was revolutionary. She felt released from the traditional view of only honouring one standard answer. She wrote,

For the first time I believe in this process, because I really see in this course that REAL knowledge is based on understanding, experience and feeling. It's so valuable.

Learning through discussion

Participants mentioned the benefits of learning through group discussion, from both personal and teaching points of view. Some members appreciated that listening to others could help them to see things from different angles, to enhance their learning from others' reflection and discussion, to learn how to present similar ideas, to analyse different viewpoints and to gain recognition for their thoughts. Yunlei further elaborated that the opportunity for group discussion was a vital element for experiential learning.

I think discussion is very vital. You led us to do the activities...let everybody try first, and then asked us to discuss the experience afterwards. It was very effective. I found it was worthwhile to spend time on thorough discussion. I will take it back to my work. Next time when I conduct a workshop, I will teach in this way...Lack of discussion limits the participants' learning. Through discussion, they can understand why we did this and that...This will become one of the important elements in my workshop design in future.

The qualities of the facilitator

Although this was not explicitly a teaching method workshop, it is an important extended pedagogical learning; as the facilitator, I too was reminded of the qualities required during teaching. Some participants documented their observation and learning of facilitation during the workshop. Like Qiling,

After experiencing the session today, I think I need to spend more time to listen to the participants in my workshop. Be patient and give enough space for them (especially in the discussion section). Furthermore, the facilitator should be the first to show a high level of engagement. This is the critical factor to lead the participants and make them feel engaged.

Zhuhui noted that he had learned that a good facilitator should be a good communicator who was expressive, attentive, and sincere. At the same time, he reflected on his current working style and wanted to make a change.

> *When I communicate with clients, I should be an attentive and active listener. As I learnt from today's workshop, the delivery of ideas should be clear to make communication effectively. I used to work casually with clients; I must improve my emotional control and create good conditions.*

Cameo 1: Minxia's change in practice

Minxia was one participant who frequently mentioned pedagogical learning. She gained her belief in the pedagogy from her personal feelings and the observation of the participants' changes in the process. She was excited and actively put the learning into practice after the training. She shared a number of snapshots to show how she was applying the new pedagogy. The positive responses she received from the clients reinforced her belief. Most importantly, she found herself being more professional. I have chosen three snapshots to demonstrate how she applied the learning through changes in her practice.

Snapshot 1: client-centred pedagogy

In a workshop for a group of workers at a social welfare centre, she was alerted by her colleagues that it was a tough group, with low motivation. She had been used to begin with simple physical exercises for ice-breaking; whereas this time, she broke the ice by touching the participants' inner feelings. She imagined and felt their working situation from their position: they were a group of hard-working social workers, whose contribution was always being neglected by the general public. She started the workshop by sharing her personal story; then gradually she invited them, via sharing their own backgrounds and hobbies, to share their feelings about their work.

> *Please step forward if you:*
>
> * *like eating fruits;*
> * *are a parent;*
> * *feel pressure at work;*
> * *feel happy at work;*
> * *feel lost at work sometimes…*

The questions Minxia chose to ask made the participants feel they were being recognised and of concern to someone. She commented on her new approach to beginning a workshop:

Through the process of asking questions, I came to feel that they really gave a lot of effort to their organisation. I said thanks to them, thanked them for their contribution to serving under-privileged people. Their silence showed this was well-received. Some participants told me there was nobody who had said thanks to them before. They had resisted and ignored previous workshops because they thought the facilitators did not understand them. So, I feel it is very important to respect people.

Her participants were highly engaged in the rest of this workshop. Minxia had put herself into their shoes, felt their emotions, and paid tribute to their efforts. This new client-based paradigm was rewarded by their appreciation.

Snapshot 2: participation and self-constructive learning

In the same workshop, the core activity was teaching the social workers how to assess a student with special needs. In the past, Minxia had used one-way, didactic pedagogy, to tell the participants what they should do. This time, she invited one participant to describe a student problem as a case, then discussed that openly with all the social workers. Through her interaction with the student, she asked the participants, 'What do you think we should do with this student?'

This is very unusual for me. I learnt it from you in the workshop. I never asked this question in my previous teaching. Before, I would directly tell them what they should do without inviting their suggestions. Now I found they actually knew their students very well. I only needed to help them think about the things they could do. They knew best about their students' needs. My imposed suggestions could not always work for them.

Minxia changed her one-way pedagogy to invite participation, engaging them as active participants instead of passive recipients. She trusted the participants' ability and honoured the knowledge they had accumulated from daily working experience. She was feeling good and satisfied with her change in practice, especially seeing that 'a tough group with low motivation' turned into 'an active engaged group'.

Snapshot 3: empowerment and collaborative learning

At the end of another workshop she conducted, Minxia changed the expert-centred method of holding a Q&A session. Instead of the facilitator as an expert giving answers, she invited participants to come out and ask their questions, and opened the space for whole-group collaborative exploration. She encouraged the participants to stand up and find their own voice. Then she invited everyone to write down their ideas and suggestions on paper. The questioner collected these, read them out, and discussed them with the group. They were also able to keep the papers for their further reference.

*I found it was a very good method. I learnt a lot from the participants.
When I used the old way to conduct this section, I became the 'big figure'
and never got a chance to learn from others…it was good also because
everybody could suggest different ways to deal with the problem, which created more possibilities.*

She was impressed by the shared learning space where the active participation
evolved. She found changing the role from being the expert to a co-learner
increased the level of acceptance by the participants as well as their learning
opportunities. She commented herself:

I felt very good. More importantly, I now feel I am more professional.

Reflective learning

There was limited explicit description from the participants about reflective
learning. Most of the participants claimed they were 'more reflective' after the
workshop but found it hard to articulate in words what exactly that meant, and
what was the content of this type of learning. Reflective capacity is an inner
quality. The setting, structure, activities, and tasks all had the potential to provide the 'reflective space' for the participants. Apart from the participants naming this kind of learning, reflection as action was embedded in the activities
and tasks in the workshop. Although the participants did not particularly
speak about their reflective learning, they did show their reflective responses
during the learning process itself. For instance, the Category Two and Three
participants made relatively less mention of reflective learning in the interview
and/or final essay; however, they did ask sophisticated reflective questions (the
reader may refer back to some of those in this chapter and the previous) during
the group discussion and in the journal. They did not talk about reflection;
they showed the act of reflection in the process.

Jingjing was a typical case. She mentioned many times that she had always
started by learning theory before experience. This training workshop was set
up on experiential learning, which she thought actually hindered her learning.

*You asked me to reflect after the experience, I didn't know how to do reflec-
tion…I participated in all the activities. Sometimes, I could not think of
anything…I participated, I experienced, but I could not reflect deeply and
only stayed at a very superficial level.*

Jingjing was in fact able to articulate some of her learning experience and
learning preference, which in one sense shows a general kind of reflection. In a
broad sense, all the types of learning analysed above involved reflective capacity. What the participants shared in applied theatre learning and generic learnings are kinds of reflective learning. Through reflection, they consolidated,

synthesised, and summarised their learning in the workshop, as well as their unsuccessful learning experiences. Reviewing these, I extrapolated the following three areas as what they thought had been of significant value to themselves:

- aspects of the workshop that helped to build reflective capacity;
- a sense of change;
- the value for themselves of being reflective.

There were three components of the workshop that the participants thought were particularly helpful to their reflective learning: the reflective journal, the teaching methods, and the interview.

Reflective journal

Most of the participants had not written a reflective journal before. They generally gave positive comments on this task and said they would recommend it to their colleagues. Most of them found it useful to note down their important feelings, thoughts, and moments after the experience.

> *The reflective journal is very special to me. It was able to help me to document what I was thinking, what I was doing and to reflect on why I had these responses…If one did not do that, one would regret it. One cannot ever recall the same feeling again.*

> (Baiyi)

The journal gave them material to reflect on the process in future. Jieyan believed that she would gain more understanding from reviewing the journal from time to time. Qiling pointed out the act of writing itself was a process of thinking.

> *The reflective journal helped me to consolidate the experience and my thoughts in each session. This was a process of reflection. It made a difference if you got a chance to write down something. It helped my mind become clearer and more systematic.*

Although the participants were not sure if they could form a writing habit after the workshop, some tried to find a way to sustain this spirit. Baiyi mentioned he would now make notes and write reminders for his next practice after each workshop he conducted. However, not every participant really understood the function of the journal, though I put instructions and a set of guiding questions on the first journal task. Some wrote very brief and short notes; some just used the journal to take notes on the procedures of different activities. Some found it difficult to document their learning through writing. Like Liliang:

> *I had lot of feelings during the activities. However, I found it very hard and did not know how to write through words in the reflective journal. I could not write.*

Reading Liliang's reflective journal, though his writing in Phases Two and Three was short and shallow, I found that what he had said was not the whole story. He did reflect on personal awareness quite deeply in Phase One, in which he still felt confident and excited about learning.

Dialogical teaching

Many participants mentioned that my choice of stepping back and not giving standard answers for all their questions effectively helped them to build reflective capacity. It gave them a space and motivated them to think independently. Jieyan expressed how this benefited her learning:

> *If you had given me more direction and provided answers, I would have thought less. I was not being reflective in the previous workshops I attended. Here, you provided me space to think and reflect. It was important. If you gave me all the concepts instead of allowing me to build them by myself, I would not remember them. The knowledge created through my own thinking process can be a resource for future practice.*

My teaching method not only influenced the participants' reflective capacity. It could also be an experience to be reflected on. Meili recognised the benefit of not being limited by being given an absolute answer, and linked this idea to thinking about her work:

> *Now I will think: will I block the children's imaginative ability if I only give them one absolute answer?*

She demonstrated her reflective capacity by asking more reflective questions:

> *It is clear that the participatory way of teaching has many benefits. The current examination-oriented education does limit the students' creativity. However, is the participatory way the best way of teaching? Is it more suitable to apply where there is an open learning objective? Is it appropriate to decide whether we use a participatory, semi-participatory or traditional way of teaching, depending on the students' stage of development?*

Interviews

Surprisingly to me, the interview was one of the methods I used which turned out to play a pedagogical role in contributing to the participants' reflective learning. The participants took those opportunities to think about and talk about learning. The interview was an act of reflection. Some participants mentioned it could give them a reflective space to consolidate the learning from the training workshop.

> *I have a strong memory of the time talking with you at interviews. This was a space for contemplation and for consolidating learning.*

(Xunxi)

The interview also provided a platform for participants to reflect on their practice. Baiyi valued this:

> *Interview is a good platform for me to consolidate my experience. I can reflect on my practice while sharing it with you. It enhances my thinking ability and affects my way of thinking.*

Sense of change after the workshop

A number of participants mentioned they got a feeling of change in thinking habits and at work. Jieyan described the reflective capacity she gained as like 'the third eye'. She was able to 'jump out' to observe herself while she was doing an activity. She compared the learning this time with her previous workshop experience.

> *I am a lazy person. Although the workshops I attended always emphasised self-awareness and self-reflection, I was still passive for change. However, in this workshop, I have gradually created a habit to become aware of myself. I unconsciously make myself alert to what I am doing and what I feel in every moment. Asking why. For a lazy person like me, this habit is a very important reward.*

Carrying this similar sense of gaining reflective capacity, participants like Anwen and Meili found an obvious change in their thinking pattern at work. They found themselves asking 'why' at work with increasing frequency, which was new to their life. Yumei said,

> *I have increased times for self-reflection and self-evaluation both at work and in life. When I meet people, I will automatically think and reflect on what they said they meant.*

Meili thought this change could make her more understanding of her clients. Both of them mentioned that their colleagues expressed positive comments on their change.

There were a few participants who mentioned that their reflective capacity could help them to make better professional judgements.

It is very important to have reflective ability. I always tell people: if we don't learn from mistakes, we will keep repeating the same fault; if we don't know there is a mistake, we can never improve.

Yunlei suggested that reflective capacity is critical to NGO workers. It could help them to learn from experience. Although she did not think she was reflective enough, the experience obtained from the training workshop gave her a guide to practice. She valued the importance of being reflective, especially in the Chinese context:

I think this ability is very important. It is very dangerous if we can only see things in black or white. It is dangerous especially, living under the thinking mode of our country's party. Being reflective is very useful.

Cameo 2: Zhuhui's reflective learning

Zhuhui described a strong sense of reflective learning after the workshop. I found his account indicated that all three of the above-mentioned areas of generic learning were involved.

Journal

When I reviewed my journal, I felt what I had written was unbelievable. The writing was unusual. The words I used were sophisticated and deep. I was able only to describe the concrete and superficial things before, but this time I could explain the abstract ideas.

Teaching method

I think the way you taught was good. If you had behaved like a traditional teacher, I would have relied on you, which would have hindered my learning. Since the beginning of this training workshop, I have been learning to think independently. When I go back to my working environment, I can still think on my own without relying on you.

Interview

I find the interview has a function of helping me to consolidate my learning and give me room for reflection. When I listened to the recording of our second interview, I felt it was quite 'painful' since you pushed me to think and reflect. You helped me to analyse and understand what I had done, to dig deep into my thoughts.

Sense of change after the training workshop

> *In the past, my thinking was very simple and superficial whereas now it is at a deeper level. I will think about why something has happened. My reflective capacity has gradually developed. I think it is good to see things thoroughly. I know how to summarise different ideas. The bad thing is sometimes I feel confused. When I sort out one problem, another problem comes up. The more I reflect, the more questions. It is still good to generate a motivating force to improve.*

The value of being reflective

> *I felt my growth used to be very flat. But gradually now, I feel my capacity has been developing like stepping up stairs…having reflective capacity helps me to improve quickly. In the past, I could only deal with problems one by one and mostly superficially. I did not know how to put the relevant issues together and find out the original cause of a problem. Now, I can do it better…*
>
> *In the past, I would take for granted all the things that happened in the activity and had no reflection after the experience. Now I will reflect on the experience and check if it matched with the objectives, the clients' needs and the rationale…*
>
> *In the past, I only wrote my report on what I saw, very simply. Now I will add in my reflection and provide alternative ideas. In the organisation's general meetings, I can now give more sophisticated suggestions. I have found my colleagues looking at me differently.*

Zhuhui's comments show how the accumulated and holistic influence from all the areas of generic knowing generated deep learning that benefited his personal capacity and professional growth. His story was typical of that holistic understanding that burgeoned among many of the participants in the workshop, though not all could articulate it so eloquently.

7 The facilitator's voice

It's all about me

At the start of the project, as I mentioned, my plan was based quite simply on two clear teaching domains, to train the participants in *applied theatre learning*, and train them in or help them develop the *generic skills* that underpin applied theatre (personal, pedagogical, and reflective skills). I also recognised that I would categorise and document the extent to which the participants' attention was focused on the facilitator, and therefore how the training was being run (not much attention from the beginners, very much more for Category Three). Almost from the outset, and more and more as the workshop progressed and deepened, I realised that the skills and capabilities of their facilitator was a third learning domain that was equally important to all these trainees – some of their comments that you have read in the last two chapters already indicate this. Accordingly, I brought to front of mind, and planning, and documentation, what had been a quite secondary research intention of mine, to research and reflect upon my own practice in the workshop. The capacities of the facilitator were just as important to the participants as they were to me, so I found myself self-consciously demonstrating myself. It was unavoidable, because it was more and more front of mind for them, and, I realised, just as crucial a part of the training as any of the applied theatre or generic skills.

They needed to know from me, as the facilitator who set up and structured the training workshop: what were the underpinning assumptions from my own theory of practice? How do I understand what I did? How had this influenced the planning and my behaviour towards them? Why was I responding to them and the training in the way I was? In fact, my own theory of practice was continuously evolving in the process. I was not fully clear about my teaching choices, even as I was making them. Gradually, through their perceptive commentary on me, and my own sustained reflective processes, I found an alignment between the workshop action and my educational theory; some of this will become evident throughout this chapter and the next.

DOI: 10.4324/9781003426387-9

Preliminaries

There was quite a lot to be done by the facilitator before we started, even after the selection process, which was vital in itself, but for many groups of trainees and their facilitators, not always so fortunately controllable as mine was.

Letter before briefing session

I made it clear to the potential participants my emphases on this way of learning and my positioning at the outset – before they came to the briefing session, so that they could make an informed decision:

> *This training workshop puts strong emphasis on the participants' reflection and documentation of their experience. For consolidating and internalising the learning, every participant has to write a journal, do some reflection and join in discussion during the course.*
>
> *The workshop is not a teaching course for experts. I position this course as a platform to co-explore the application of applied theatre between facilitator and participants. I will share my knowledge and so will you, sharing your working experience and needs. With support from the group, I hope you can become a reflective practitioner.*

First interview

In the interview before the training workshop started, I expressed what I expected of their attitude to learning. The following main points, raised during these preliminary interviews, together illustrate my personal theory of learning, so I was able to attempt to reinforce them throughout.

Respect for different paces of learning (especially for beginners)

(To Anwen) Learning is a personal activity. It starts at your own pace. It doesn't matter if you walk on a different path. No need to make comparisons. It is not about who is better than whom. Doesn't matter! Because everyone is independent and unique. For me, I am also new to the group. I have never worked with you guys before. Everyone is different. Every time is our first time.

Independent learning

(To Tianxin) We have to build our way of learning internally. If you can build your own system for learning in these few months, you can go further after this training workshop. Learning is a lifelong matter.

Learning from others

*(To Baiyi) I hope everybody in this training workshop can share their expe-
rience and ideas on applied theatre with each other. We will explore the
activities together. We can discuss the possibilities for applying the activities, to dig deep into their meaning. I hope we are a learning community.*

*(To Qiling) We are a community. Everyone has different experiences
and can inspire each other. I am not the only one you can talk to. You may
discuss and explore with any one of our group members…Everyone may
have a different interpretation of an activity. So, it will be a chance for you
to synthesise different ideas.*

Encouraging reflection

*(To Zhuhui) It is critical that you can train your mind to be more reflective.
You told me you want to be more professional. I think the critical quality in
being a professional is reflective ability.*

Encouraging experienced participants to dig deep

*(To Tianxin) I would like to encourage you to achieve a higher level of
learning. Since you have learnt some activities before, this time you have the
opportunity to observe how a beginner starts to learn the activities. At your
level, I will challenge you to dig deep into the understanding you already
have of the form and take note carefully of the development process of the
new learners.*

Structuring the training workshop

I chose to start the training workshop by teaching theatre of the oppressed
because the games, exercises, and activities provided direct opportunities for
self-exploration. I would be able to use participants' personal material, connecting with their inner feelings. I would become aware of their personal
choices and thoughts about different issues, and of their relationships to others. Then, process drama in Phase Two altered the experience to explore the
self and others through sustained fictional roles. Gradually, by Phase Three,
the participants were given increasing power to make decisions about the top-
ics/issues they wanted to explore using applied theatre themselves (at least the
forms of forum theatre, process drama and participatory theatre). They had to
reflect on their main concern at that moment of life and put it into action.

Selecting topics

In Phase One, through demonstrating the theatre of the oppressed (TO) exercises and activities, I purposely put one of my teaching emphases on helping the
participants reflect on their current condition. I also encouraged them to actively

think about what they wanted to explore and which issues most concerned them at this moment, and to share their views on different issues in action. Although TO, by its nature, embeds the potential for self-exploration, this genre is still open for the facilitator to direct the participants' focus of learning. For example, when I introduced image theatre, I chose to ask the participants to create images about their happy and unhappy moments, about what happened in their recent lives, about stories of personal struggles, etc. Though I chose some of the foci for their learning, I took care not to limit the discussion and reflection, which was also a space for them to practise mindful awareness. The following extract shows the participants sharing in reflection and their new awareness of different concerns after the exercise on making happy and unhappy images:

YM: *What do you feel about the exercise?*

P1: *From feeling relaxed to feeling tense.*

P2: *I find happiness is much easier to empathise with than unhappiness.*

P3: *I have a thought. If we first make an unhappy image before the happy image, there might be a therapeutic effect.*

P4: *I find the physical condition can affect emotion.*

YM: *Did it affect you in the process?*

P4: *When I made the happy image, I felt more positive, whereas the unhappy image made me feel unhappy.*

P5: *At the moment when everybody was dismissed, I felt happiness could be shared but unhappiness only belonged to myself.*

YM: *So according to your observation, was it like your real-life situation?*

P5: *Oh...I think it is.*

P6: *I find I don't really know my body. I spent quite a long time thinking of making the images. I didn't really pay attention to my physical status.*

Asking the right questions

Apart from choosing topics to raise awareness, I always asked follow-up questions to help the participants think deeply. I used the 'shaking hands' activity in Phase One as an example. It is a common warm-up activity in applied theatre workshops. Some facilitators use it as a mild and non-threatening physical contact game to start a workshop. I shared this objective and then added my own agenda. I did this activity twice in different versions. In the sharing after version one, participants listened to the diversity of responses. Each expression showed a different individual personality. Members started to build connections with each other. I saw my role as a reminder to the participants to go back to their own inner feelings and to encourage them to be mindfully aware of what they felt in the process.

YM: *What did you feel during the activity?*

P1:   *I didn't really know who I shook hands with.*

YM: *So, this was your feeling in the process? Anyone has a different feeling?*

P2:   *I shook hands with some people twice; but some not at all.*

P3:   *I feel very artificial.*

YM: *What made you feel artificial?*

P3:   *Too quick.*

P4:   *I felt the process was very messy. Shaking hands was like completing a task.*

YM: *What was this feeling of completing a task like?*

P4:   *I could not feel anything. I did not even know whose hands I shook with.*

P5:   *There were some hands holding me with a friendly force. I had a sense of connection.*

P2:   *Someone held me with both hands.*

YM: *So, was there any difference for people holding you with one hand or both hands?*

P2:   *Holding with both hands made me feel very warm and seemed to say: 'I miss you so much'.*

P6:   *I felt people just wanted to finish a task.*

YM: *So, did you treat the exercise as finishing a task?*

P6:   *No, I didn't. If I had done that, it would have made the exercise meaningless.*

P7:   *I was different from you. I did shake hands with my heart and said 'Hello' to everyone I met during the process.*

YM: *Does anyone remember if you shook hands with P7? Did you feel her sincerity?* (some nod)

P8:   *I found someone who was very creative and found an efficient way to shake everybody's hands within a short time.* (shows this way of handshaking)

P9:   *I originally used my right hand. When I saw someone using an efficient way, I hesitated about whether I needed to change my way.*

P10:   *I specially approached the people I did not know before.*

P11:   *I felt very happy to meet many old faces and new friends.*

YM: *Anyone who shook hands with P11?* (many people put hands up)

YM: *Did you feel her happiness?* (many people nod)

The second time, I invited the participants to associate the experience with their real-life situation. I asked questions to heighten their self-observation. Though their answers were short, in this first activity of the training workshop I wanted to subtly link reflection to their real-life situation. Here are extracts of two participants' responses:

P12:   *I got lost! In the beginning, I was holding hands with two persons. When everybody had finished shaking hands with everybody else, there was a moment with no hand holding mine. I did not know what to do.*

YM: *Do you always feel like this in life? Feeling lost when something suddenly disappears.*

P12:   *Yes, yes...*

YM: *Do you always have this experience?*

P12:   *It usually happens at work. I sometimes get lost...having this feeling.*

P13:   *I found myself always standing at the edge of the circle.*

YM: *Did you shake any hands?*

P13:   *Yes. When I was nearly finished, I chose to stand at the edge. After a while, I hesitated. Then I thought I should stand inside the circle.*

YM: *What did you feel when you stood at the edge?*

P13:   *I felt many people were very active and passionate. I also saw some people who treated the activity as merely a task.*

YM: *So, in your life, do you always choose to stand at the edge?*

P13:   *Yes, always...*

YM: *Do you think it is the most comfortable position for you?*

P13:   *True. Yes!*

I encouraged them to be aware of their feelings and turn them into words. Several of the activities in Phase One, such as mirroring and sculpting exercises, rainbow of desire, cops-in-the-head, had a similar focus: to raise mindful awareness, and connect inner feelings to reflection-in-action.

In Phase Two, process drama, my selection of lesson plans was based on sharing a variety of process dramas with various lengths and structures, using diverse sets of conventions and pre-texts, and different age targets. I hoped the selections offered a wide range of inputs for reflection after action. The participants accumulated their experience in five process dramas as a source for them to think about both the general principles and the specifics of process drama. The experiential period gave them a foundation to construct learning in the reflective processes.

In this phase, selecting roles for participants in the different process dramas was not my priority in the lesson planning. I invited participants to share their feelings in-between the episodes in each drama. I also asked questions to link their feelings back to their own lives after the dramas. To a certain extent, I wanted to keep the custom of encouraging awareness of the relationship between drama and life. Through the in-role and out-of-role reflection, I hoped to help participants to enhance their self-awareness by articulating their feelings and thoughts.

This extract is an example of in-role shared reflection in the process drama *Green Children* – a well-used drama structure popularised by Julie Dunn (2022) – after they had role-played one of the green children with a non-green friend, in pairs:

YM: *What did you feel in this episode?*
P1:   *I did not understand what he meant. I felt very nervous and worried by his emotion.*
P2:   *I could feel his friendliness.*
YM: *So, did you increase the level of acceptance during the process?*
P2:   *(nod) Yes.*
P3:   *When he first came in, he touched me gently. I felt he was nice and friendly.*
P4:   *He showed me many different kinds of green things. This…and that…although I did not understand his language, I could feel he was kind to me.*
P5:   *He kept forcing me to eat things.*
YM: *What did you feel when he forced you to eat?*
P5:   *In the beginning, I felt he was nice. But gradually, I felt helpless because he kept giving me things I didn't want.*

The reflective journal

A journal is a vehicle for reflection. It is a private space for the participants to organise learning from their own point of view after the experience. Many researchers and facilitators use reflective journals, but not always with clear or common purposes. To clarify my own thinking, I followed the advice of Jennifer Moon (1999, 188–194) on the purposes of writing journals, which I think is worth quoting in full, as it formed a major part of my planning. These include:

• To deepen the quality of learning, in the form of critical thinking or developing a questioning attitude
• To enable learners to understand their own learning process
• To increase active involvement in learning and personal ownership of learning
• To enhance professional practice or the professional self in practice
• To enhance the personal valuing of the self towards self-empowerment

- To enhance creativity by making better use of intuitive understanding
- To free up writing and the representation of learning
- To provide an alternative 'voice' for those not good at expressing themselves
- To foster reflective and creative interaction in a group

This list equally defined my whole objective for promoting independent and self-constructive learning in this training workshop. The participants documented the things they felt most interested in and their main concerns during the learning process. The entries could also be a record of growth and of honouring an individual experience. Most importantly, the participants were encouraged to be active learners and had an opportunity to find their own voice in the process.

The following note I put on the first page of the journal to share my own thoughts about the functions of the journal with the participants, and as a reminder of why they were writing it.

We believe our wisdom grows from wholeheartedly living in the experience, attentive observation and full reflection. Learning can be gained if you have enough courage to face yourself as you really are.

We start from where we are, not following others.

We keep our own pace and walk towards the inner depth of mind.

We hope this journal as a private document can create a space for personal development, for contemplation after action. It can help us to organise, extend and consolidate the learning after the experience.

We hope this learning record can accompany you and bring you a new perspective to dialogue with yourself, others and the world.

Every small step is like a drop of water everyday accumulating to build your understanding. Only you can open the door of learning, provided that you are taking it seriously enough. No one can replace you for learning, only YOU can do it for yourself!

A warm reminder during the writing (adapted from Moon, 1999:102):

- *Let words flow – write about whatever is at the top of your mind; uncensored, no polish is needed; ideas will come before you know it and surprise you.*
- *Use your own words – put your name on things, not what others say; be honest, say what you feel and think.*
- *Dig deeper – urge yourself to keep digging deeper and deeper so that you can understand and use your understanding. Link to your authentic feeling and thinking. Ask yourself questions about the experience and thoughts generated, to search your 'truth' through linking with your inner self.*

There was no fixed format to record the experience. To stimulate their thinking, I did provide some guiding questions as a reference to the participants. The participants wrote their journal at the end of each session. At the final session in Phases One and Two, they were given time to review their earlier entries and summarise the central concern and issue they felt most important from reading the pages.

Collective reflection on action

The group gathered together at the beginning of every session. The main purpose of these sessions was to encourage the sharing of feelings, thoughts, and questions raised in the previous session. To create a space for the participants to express and connect with each other, I usually started by checking-in with all the participants and asking them to reflect on their week.

> *I would like you to take this moment as a space, a stage for your own to share and express the feelings of your week by creating an image. Let's begin with sharing your feelings at this moment. To express is an action. I invite you to come out and sit on this stool during your sharing.*

I wanted to encourage every participant from the start to be aware of their own personal feelings and practise connecting those with others. At the beginning of a session, I started by inviting the participants to be aware of the place they chose to sit, and think about the relationship between self and space, about space and people. From the physical distance to mental distance, I wanted the participants to reflect on their relationships with others. I intended to create a platform for social communication. Through encouraging the participants to express themselves to others, I hoped for them to gain self-confidence and at the same time to strengthen the connections in the group. The participants were able to learn from seeing others' ways of interaction and expression. I thought creating a culture of connection, sharing, and acceptance would be helpful to enhance reflection for learning in the group.

The focus of the discussion would follow the flow of the participants' concerns as well as the reflective questions I posed. In Phase One, the discussion usually started with me inviting the participants to talk about their experience. They shared their thoughts on what had given them strong feelings. To begin with the participants' concerns is crucial. I believed that they could not learn everything in one training workshop, and so it was more important to allow a space for their own learning. They were encouraged to construct their learning from 'where they were' and from their own needs and interests. Furthermore, they raised their concerns publicly. The personal sharing was no longer personal. It provided an opportunity for collective reflection and learning.

In Phase Two, I asked structured questions as part of my teaching.

- *So far, for you, what is applied theatre?*
- *What do you think about the features of process drama?*
- *What do you think are the learning objectives in each lesson plan?*
- *What is/are your personal learning point(s) from the micro-teaching?*

I posed the questions to help the participants to reflect and make sense of the experience. The participants would be invited to share their personal thoughts either in whole-group discussion or in small groups before sharing them publicly. As if they were drawing a picture collectively, everyone contributed part of it and built on their understanding. They practised articulating their experience into words; at the same time, they listened to others' thoughts and feelings. Generally, I did not limit the group time. I gave as much time as possible for the discussion, because I thought it was important to provide space for thinking, expressing thoughts, asking questions and talking to each other.

I played several roles during the group time: facilitator, questioner, observer, researcher, participant, and teacher. I put the emphasis on encouraging the participants to focus on self-awareness, asking them: what they felt about the experience, what they thought, and why they thought what they thought. I would sometimes share examples, experiences, and stories from my work. When they asked me questions, most of the time, I held back my opinion and was reluctant to give a 'standard answer'. I would rather say,

- *Good...jot down your findings. Keep exploring them.*
- *I have no answers. I encourage you to continue to find out more, searching from your practice.*

Or I would ask follow-up questions to help them think below the surface:

- *Can you imagine why you have these kinds of feeling?*
- *What did you do at that moment of difficulty? How did you cope with it?*
- *Do you know why you are afraid of showing your body in the mirror exercise?*

Or I would seek the opinions of other group members:

- *Is there anybody who can offer a suggestion for solving this problem? Does anyone share his/her feeling?*

From time to time, instead of giving 'the answer', I encouraged the importance of mindful awareness when they had doubts about learning.

We learn at every moment. Everyone has their own pace. Some learn things fast, whereas others need more time. There may be an inner voice that says, 'I am a slow learner. Other members have more experience. I am good at nothing'...Therefore, please give yourself space to learn about yourself. You may find you are a person who fears standing in front of people. You may find you like to be the best and perfect. It is important to reflect and ask yourself, 'Where have these ideas come from?' Have they come from yourself? Or have they come from the facilitator's pressure?...I think the awareness is quite crucial. This is a good starting point.

(From my opening remarks, Week 1)

I would share my personal theory of learning about applied theatre in the group time to explain my teaching methods.

> *I am hoping to provide you with a method of sustainable learning. Actually, I also learn this way. You need to practise applied theatre in your own context independently. No one will be available to help you all the time.*

Participants' responses

In expressing what the participants valued in the training, my teaching method was a theme they mentioned often. They mentioned aspects that aligned with what I intended to do according to my personal learning theory. Although I did not take my educative influence for granted, what they described and how they responded to their learning experience can provide a cross-reference for examining my practice. In this section, after delineating the themes and sub-themes, I am once more allowing these, in the main, highly articulate students to speak with their own words, rather than paraphrasing and editorialising, as their words resonate together to create a natural synthesis. I shall be analysing and extrapolating from their testimony in the next chapters. Most of the participants described my teaching and learning method by comparing it to traditional education and their own previous learning experiences. They found our way very different. They made sense of this by finding what was new to them.

Self-constructive learning and teacher–learner relationship

> *In my past, everything would be given a definition. I would be told what should be learnt, very clearly. Then, teacher would give you some examples to help you understand the application. However, this time, we must learn by ourselves…we need to experience and feel. Then we must examine the contents to construct our own meaning.*
>
> (Luping)

This is a typical response. They further explained the unexpected teacher–student relationship in this training workshop.

> *I am used to thinking the teacher should answer all questions. However, the way you teach – pushing us to think, to find out the answers – is very different from my knowledge of the role of teacher.*
>
> (Yunlei)

They found they could not depend on me.

> *I totally relied on my teacher in the past. If I had a question, the teacher would tell me the answer or give me a very concrete guideline to find the*

answer. However, I cannot think you will do the same in this workshop. I have to play an active role to internalise the learning in the process.

(Jingjing)

They even used the mother–child relationship to describe their past learning.

We are used to putting the focus on the teacher: as a child waits for their mother for feeding. But 'the mother' here is not prepared to feed us at all.

(Xunxi)

Documentation and reflection

I take many notes. And I have to think about them. I found this time that I take writing my journal very seriously. I have never written that much before. This will affect my learning. In my previous performing arts workshops, I never documented my feelings about the dance and singing I participated in. This time, I want to write about it all.

(Baiyi)

Learning from experience

I find it is a very attractive and interesting way of learning. People said we study knowledge to apply it. This time, we play to learn. We absorb the knowledge from playing games.

(Liliang)

We must move our bodies and participate in this workshop – very different to traditional Chinese education There were only two PPT presentations throughout, and also very few teacher lectures; we mainly participated in drama, discussion and sharing.

(Qiling)

Learning from others

This time every participant shares their experience and knowledge. I have a very strong feeling that we have been constructing our learning all together this time. I find this workshop makes everybody visible. In my past learning, the participants were invisible, and they spoke not even a sentence, just like a passer-by. But here, everybody stands out.

(Luping)

Freedom in the learning process

> *Here, I feel everybody can be close and friendly to each other. In previous workshops and classes I have attended, the teacher always sat in the front, and we all sat in rows facing the blackboard – whereas here we can be free to express ourselves.*
>
> (Xinhong)

> *I can lie on the floor in this training workshop. I feel very comfortable.*
> (Anwen)

There were two stages in their responses to these novel learning methods.

Struggling stage

Many participants expressed that they found the beginning phase was 'painful' and 'tiring' since they had to do a lot of reflection and rely on self-constructive learning, which was unfamiliar for them. They were confused and did not know how to learn and what to learn in the process. They expected me as an expert teacher to provide definitions and explanations after the activities. They had a particular function of 'teacher' in mind and thought this was my job to provide teaching for their understanding. I was the one to set up the learning agenda and summarise the points for learning at the end of the session. Their struggles created tensions during the group time. Some participants requested me to reduce the discussion time and adjust my teaching method.

> *If this is a general workshop, the discussion can be that long. However, this is a trainer-training workshop. I think Yi-man should summarise the main points for our learning after just a short sharing among the participants. This is very important to let me understand every learning objective for each activity…I think it is more important to be directly told by the teacher.*
>
> (Zhangnan)

Although some participants like Zhangnan complained about the long discussion wasting time, not everyone agreed.

> *I agree to keep the long discussion time. Since this is the beginning phase of the training workshop, we have just started to come together as learners. Everybody has a different learning experience and level of acceptance. If there is only limited discussion time, people with more experience are likely to dominate the time. Some people may have no opportunity to express themselves. Then we have no way to feel other people, to understand the questions people have. I think it is good to put a slow pace on discussion.*
>
> (Tianxin)

The discussion makes me learn to be patient. I find learning nowadays is like a fast-food culture. Everything should be quick and efficient. No one cares whether you can learn it or not…I think a real education should accept people's differences. Be patient. It is very basic. If you cannot do this, it is not going to be useful even if you have learnt a number of skills.

(Baiyi)

Adapting stage

Though the unfamiliar learning experience made some participants struggle and feel uncomfortable, I insisted on this teaching method because I thought this pain was necessary for everybody to adapt to our new way of learning. I did not ignore their feelings. I encouraged them to connect to their inner feelings and stick to their own pace of learning. I also responded to their need for 'information feeding' by setting up a blog on the internet. I kept my style of teaching, but I agreed to put learning materials online for their reference. For Zhaofeng the consistency of this way of teaching was important to her.

It is very important for you not giving the answer. One day, if you change your style and give me the answer, it may break down my constructive learning process.

According to my observation, the participants gradually adapted to the learning method by the end of Phase One, with less tension and more focus on participating in the group discussions. They still had their doubts and confusions, but they were willing to adapt. Since they realised they could not totally rely on me, they started to seek their own learning methods. Jieyan recognised the benefit:

If you stepped out more in the front or led more in the process, I would have less opportunity to think and learn less. The space you created for my reflection and thinking was very important. If you gave me the concepts, I would not have any ownership…Now when I think of using applied theatre activities, the reflection I came across during the training workshop has left a guide to remind me.

Anwen mentioned that the emphasis on reflection and mindful awareness in the process provoked her thinking.

From learning in primary school to university, I had never actively thought 'why things happened like this and that'. Never. Because I thought things had their fixed form. I had never been aware of my inner feelings and my needs at a deeper level. I had never asked what I was thinking. This time, I will feel what I feel, ask why I have this feeling, why I behave like this…

Promoting independent and self-constructive learning helped the participants to become active learners:

> *Although I had the urge for an answer, sometimes the questions hanging in the air made me think more deeply. The questions in my mind motivated me to seek the answer. If I had been given an answer, I would not have had the drive to seek the answer in the learning process.*

(Qiling)

Most of the participants found learning benefits from this way of learning. Zhaofeng described having a chance to construct her own knowledge was like a 'liberation' and 'revolution' to her. Change from the struggling stage to the adapting stage evolved both during and following the workshops. Tianxin gradually changed her attitude about the absence of standard answers. In Phase One, she mentioned it was necessary to have standard answers for learning. At the end of Phase Two, she said in group time,

> *Although I do not really look for an answer, I do hope to learn more from the teacher's own experience…So, I feel uncomfortable every time when I ask a question. I want to listen to your (the teacher's) past experience as my reference…I can have no standard answer, but I need a point of reference.*

After the workshop was over, she had a more sophisticated reflection on getting a standard answer.

> *I find there is no standard answer for many things. We can therefore have more space…I have received 20 years of black-and-white education. In these three months, I have learnt about exploration, possibilities…I used to think you would tell me 'what applied theatre is'. I expected you would tell me the function of every activity, and who we can apply it to. I thought you would give me clear guidance. But you didn't. For a period of time, I thought I could not find useful answers because there was no guidance…Gradually, I started to question the standard answer: is there only one answer? Only one standard function? Now I think you have to use applied theatre differently with different groups of participants. One way of application may not be suitable to all groups. I think this learning is more important than learning about standard answers.*

My teaching method drove some participants to reflect on the nature of learning. For example, Yunlei compared the new experience with the traditional education she had received.

> *The education I received emphasised 'Gao, Da, Quan' – we had to model our heroes who are the strongest, greatest, flawless and perfect. Working in a community, no matter whether in a training course, workshop, discussion*

seminar or internal meeting, we have had only black or white, right or wrong. Now, you always tell us there is 'no full stop' in learning. You mentioned the space for possibilities, creating possibilities. This gives me a lot to reflect on. When I lead a group next time, I will pay more attention to the teaching I deliver, the words I say and the things I do. I will think from different angles.

(Yunlei)

Some changed their preferred way of learning after our workshop.

I am currently attending a mime workshop. When I compare that way of teaching with our workshop I find that I like your way of teaching. Although it was a painful process because you did not give us answers and we had to find our own, it was actually a very good way to learn. I like this complex process.

(Qiling)

I now compare our teaching method with any course I attend. On one occasion when I met a didactic teacher, I felt very uncomfortable.

(Luping)

Learning difficulties

Although almost all the participants mentioned that they appreciated my teaching method, there were four participants who admitted that they had learning difficulties throughout the course. Two main difficulties they noted.

Beginners need more guidance on new ways of learning. They need external support to give them ideas on what to think, how to reflect.

I am a beginner and I need more guidance. I am not like the smart students. I don't fully understand what you are talking about. I tried my best to think by myself and consulted other participants to help my understanding.

(Xinhong)

They relied strongly on their existing learning habits and found it hard to adapt to new ways of learning.

Not giving answers did limit my learning. You know the final destination, but you keep telling me to run to the end. Never-ending discussion...But I don't really have the ability to organise different ideas, so I needed your suggestions. You summarised with many different possibilities. It was at least better than giving no answer.

(Xunxi)

This teaching method blocked my learning. I know I need to learn theory before practice. I need to make everything clear before I can move. It is easier for me to learn if I have been given a clear direction...Yes, not everything has an answer. But I still hope someone can give me an answer.

(Jingjing)

Xunxi and Jingjing were two of those who recognised their ongoing learning difficulties during the course. It did not diminish their interest in trying out applied theatre strategies in their work. In the interview after the workshop, they mentioned their confidence in the effectiveness of the methods and were thinking about potential opportunities to integrate it at work.

Postscript to the project: 10 years on, what lives on?

Ten years have passed since the training workshop. As the facilitator, of course I was very interested to revisit the participants and trace whether their applied theatre training had left any lasting impact on them – and if so, what. I sent a message to invite anyone who wanted, to have an interview with me. Researchers who are familiar with longitudinal witness follow-ups will know how hard it is to get any responses after such a long time, so I did not have high expectations. My first surprise was that I received 14 responses (6 from Category One, 6 from Category Two and both the Category Three participants). I prepared the following questions to ask every participant:

- What is your current job?
- What skills do you use currently in your work?
- What do you remember about the training workshop 10 years ago?
- What kinds of skills and/or techniques that you learned in the workshop are you still using?
- What lasting influence has the workshop had on you?

In general terms, there were few significant differences among all the respondents. What they mostly still remember about the workshop was my facilitation and the ways of learning we used, like open discussion, encouraging reflection, no standard answers, self-constructive and collective learning. Then they tended to talk about their memories of their interactions with their fellow participants and the people with whom they worked together to create the participatory theatre. Some mentioned the genres that we covered in the course, or the lesson plans they liked. Quite a number of them talked about the significant moments for some individuals that they remembered, or some specific whole-group activities. However, it is interesting, and perhaps unsurprising, to note from these responses how the degree of job relevancy affected the continued application of applied theatre differently for the participants from our three categories of experience.

Category One

Job relevance is the first and most direct criterion for the Category One participants. Meili, Chenyu, Anwen, and Zhangnan have changed their jobs to a different NGO or even changed their profession. They find themselves rarely able to use applied theatre in their current workplace. Their lack of practice makes the skills and techniques they learned in the workshop seem distant and even unnecessary.

This is very different for Zhuhui and Minxia, who still work at the same NGO as when they attended the training workshop. They are able to keep ongoing practice in their daily work. Applied theatre has become among their indispensable job skills and techniques. Zhuhui, who is now a main leader in the small workers' group, passionately integrates applied theatre techniques like image theatre, forum theatre, and theatre-in-education in his working life. He treasures how effectively the applied theatre can help his workers visualise their life and work situations; facilitate their own clients to reflect on and discuss their issues; and, most importantly, to care for each other. Zhuhui actively seeks collaboration from other training workshop participants and funding to support his work with factory workers, though this is not always smooth going. Although he consistently lacks resources for implementation, applied theatre does provide for him a means for his workers to be empathetically heard, and to release their stress in the theatrical setting. It offers them a new perspective on their circumstances, leading to positive changes. The repeated benefits experienced and expressed by his clients reinforce Zhuhui's determination and commitment to continue practising applied theatre as a form of support to his work.

Minxia still works in the same charitable organisation catering for the needs of mentally disabled children and adults. But she has also been appointed as the artistic director of an arts troupe within her organisation, to provide arts education support to all her colleagues and clients. She had trained as an arts teacher before she joined the workshop. After the training, she was able to integrate the new skills and techniques to diversify her existing practice. Although she has not elected to use many of the techniques, she has kept practising a few skills, and now she has more confidence, which reinforces the benefits of applied theatre to her clients.

It seems that for Category One participants, continued practice is the key to sustaining their learning.

Category Two

Job relevance is not a critical factor for the Category Two participants, as I mentioned in the previous chapter. These participants are independent, and they use applied theatre regardless of the nature of their job. Most of the respondents in this category have embarked on a path of independent development in their careers. Jieyan has becomes a facilitation trainer. Shuxi quit his NGO – which promoted civic society – and has established his own LGBTI concern group. Luping has moved into Waldorf education. Zhaofeng has changed to work in various women's organisations. Through ongoing learning over the course of ten years, they have all, with one exception, equipped themselves with various work strategies, of which applied theatre is just one set. It is a tool to be used or not, depending on the situation. When needed, they will employ it, but they do not consider it a core strategy for their jobs. The startling exception is one Category Two participant, Qishan, who had appeared to be one of the least involved of the participants: 'like a distant observer in the workshop', I had thought, and one of the very few not already mentioned in their quoted comments in the above chapters. Since the training workshop, Qishan has established her own applied theatre group. She chose to further develop her applied theatre knowledge with more training in drama education, as well as playback theatre and drama therapy (two widely used forms of applied theatre she did not learn in my workshop). Obviously a very deep and reflective silent listener!

Category Three

Both Baiyi and Tianxin still appreciate that the training workshop strengthened their confidence and commitment to being a professional theatre practitioner. They mentioned, as they had in their exit interviews 10 years previously, that the workshop had equipped them with significant pedagogy, skills, and techniques for them become applied theatre professionals. Baiyi resigned his job at an NGO after the training workshop, and works as a full-time practitioner. Tianxin quit her job in a commercial firm and focused on developing her career as an applied theatre freelancer. Both still very actively practise in the field and have built a reputation for themselves through the years, working with different social and commercial partners. They have created their own signature programs and continue to learn from their practice. We have a name for this in Chapter 10!

Internalising the impacts...

All the respondents mentioned that the impact that truly remains with them is in the realm of generic capacities, such as reflective ability, opening up to people and work, empathetic understanding, sharing of power, dialogic learning, self-awareness and personal growth, and the facilitator's influence. Although not all of them can count on using every or even any kind of applied theatre in their work, every one of them reaffirms how much of the generic learning from the workshop they have now internalised in their lives. What surprises me is the lasting impact of the generic learning, in terms of changing not only their ways of working with co-workers and clients, but also their ways of living. Most of the respondents shared with me how they apply the openness, empathic understanding, and reflective mind, to deal with their daily relationships with family members and friends.

Segue

These three chapters, with their intelligent, frank, and nuanced comments, have been placed here, and at some length (though only a fraction of all the feedback and data), because they are essential to fully understanding the insights and understandings that as facilitator – and as co-writer – we grasped about the real impact and effects of applied theatre on a very diverse group of participants. Just as important, those participants nearly all found and articulated new depths of understanding about themselves and how to be more reflective, resilient, and generous in their professional and sometimes personal lives. Working in NGOs, all of the participants found a need, and most of them had some opportunity, to implement applied theatre with their own even more divergent consumers and clients.

The following chapters will delve down into the theoretical and practical conclusions and insights all this testimony has given us, to provide pointers towards creating some guidelines to help trainers and facilitators in applied theatre, and more widely across human services.

References

Dunn, J. (2022). The *Green Children* drama. In J. O'Toole & J. Dunn (Eds.), *Pretending to learn: Teaching drama in the primary and middle years* (3rd ed., pp. 195–212). Thorpe-Bowker.

Moon, J. (1999). *Reflection in learning and professional development: Theory and practice*. London: Routledge.

Part III

Applied theatre training

How to and why

Part III

Applied theatre training

How to and why

8 The art of the facilitator

Preamble

The previous chapter showed how pivotal to any human services highly skilled trainers are, and particularly practical workshop facilitators in the field who find themselves leading applied theatre programs in any profession or community.

With all her personal experience and minute examination of herself and her participants, and their rich response input, Yi-Man was uniquely placed to lead us in developing some trustworthy guidelines for applied theatre trainers and especially those facilitators, who are commonly, to some degree, in situations where their own training for their position has been somewhat haphazard, non-existent, focused on something else or picked up on the job.

So, this last section of the book is devoted to providing you, the readers, with those guidelines, hoping that they prove of as much practical value, and give you as much insight into this complex, and at its best dazzlingly effective, art form, as it has given both of us. With this hope, we are changing the address to let the book speak directly to you.

This too is why we are starting our guidelines with some tips for the facilitator, ever the prime mover!

Facilitator: nurse or Svengali?

Practitioners in any human services field, or its training, share a common body of explicit professional knowledge, but we are also different from one another as we bring in our own experiences and perspectives to our work, and our styles of operation. This certainly applies to facilitators and trainers in applied theatre: each of you has your own perspectives and understanding of applied theatre and how it might be learnt. These then must be blended with the objective norms, the traditions, conventions, and specialist knowledge of applied theatre practice, and whatever genre is chosen, as well as those of the particular expectations of whatever human or community context your applied theatre will be applied to. The subjectivity factors for you, the facilitator, must include: your understanding and selecting of the genres; your own embodiment of the practice and the pedagogy; and your personal theories and practice, in planning and applying applied theatre teaching and learning.

DOI: 10.4324/9781003426387-11

These are of course interwoven, as in all human services training contexts. The trainer's understanding of the theory and practice guides your selection of the content, and how that is manifested and managed in the training. In the case of applied theatre, this includes the choice of genre. These are factors that will influence the learning. You are the key agent to bridge the gap between the participants and the practice. Alongside teaching techniques and knowledge, you need to focus on nurturing the participants' personal and social attributes that will sustain their learning and practice. This is particularly true for applied theatre, because of the fragmented, changing, and volatile nature of much learning in the field, and in the working contexts of many services to which it is being applied. Applied theatre learners, especially those working in a community context, have to equip themselves to be independent and self-constructive learners, so as to be able to scaffold their learning in what are invariably piece-meal learning situations.

Consequently, you have to use the living culture of the trainees as the soil at the base of any training program, to allow them to grow into independence. Two attributes, *mindful awareness* and *reflection*, are good guiding principles for the teaching decisions made in training workshops, in planning, instruction, and facilitation: the key capacities that will support and sustain the trainees' learning, both during and after the training. A little at a time throughout the training process, you need to consciously bring in the concepts of promoting mindful awareness and reflection. As planner or curriculum designer you will structure the training with that intent, in setting up the teaching content, order of genres, other assigned tasks and activities, and selected topics. Through this ordered process, you can structure the context to allow the participants to exercise and practise those concepts for themselves.

Yi-Man's participants came to understand and to articulate the benefits, such as trainees needing to emerge from their training able to describe aspects of the learning culture, such as learning from each other, people-centredness, a sense of freedom, and reflective and dialogical learning. The emphasis on mindful awareness impacts directly on participants' *personal learning*, which also contributes to promoting the participants' *reflective learning*. Mindful awareness is similar to the capacity to feel throughout the training process that they are consciously being and doing. This capacity is the food for reflection. The deeper the feeling of self and others, the deeper the reflection. As David Wright reminds us,

> without feeling, there is no need for reflection – thus without feeling, there is no consciousness.
>
> (2005: page unnumbered)

Your emphasis on building the capacity to feel mindfully contributes to the learner's capacity to reflect throughout the learning process. They are complementary to one another. Therefore, those capacities cannot be taken for granted, but learning through applied theatre provides rich potential for them.

The extra layer of the facilitator's own theory of practice also plays a critical role in directing the focus of learning. So that is also a part of the design which must be explicitly acknowledged.

Knowledge and competing cultures

In the next chapter, when we address the different kinds of learning/knowing generated by the applied theatre learning experience in general, the reader may discern Yi-Man's facilitator's fingerprints on the individual choices that she gradually introduced. She consciously built a structure of learning and living culture to enrich the participants' mindful awareness across the applied theatre learning experience. In every kind of human and social knowing/learning, it is necessary to help the participants to be fully present: to be aware of what is happening in their mind and body as well as the responses of those around. It is necessary to work internally with the participants, as well as externally, to sharpen their sensitivity for further reflection. Good applied theatre practice will bring awareness to the participants, but it also requires you to place a focus on manifesting it yourself during the learning process.

In nurturing the participants into being independent and self-constructive learners, mindful awareness is just the first step. This in turn goes along with promoting reflection. However, you may find this provides you and them with a significant challenge to overcome, due to a cultural struggle. In Yi-Man's study, the cultural parameters of the Chinese participants meant that they came with different perceptions of and expectations for teaching and learning from the basically Western-origin applied theatre pedagogy – or any conception of mindful awareness. Learning mindful awareness and reflection must be backed up by changes in the learning culture of the group, even if they are uncomfortable for them.

You are the person who initiates and models the way of teaching and learning, which must in the end synch with the trainees' own original culture and beliefs about learning and teaching. Applied theatre norms include that both teaching and learning are embodied, constructive, and experiential; the facilitator will usually play a role as a member in the group, rather than the sole and separate transmitter of information and instructor. This demands that the training leaves space for participants to learn from their own experience, awareness, reflection and from each other.

Yi-Man did not expect, in Phase One of her workshop, that some participants would express discomfort and confusion when asked to learn through this experimental, reflective, collaborative approach. Some responded reluctantly. They discussed their struggles and asked her for more teacher's talk and standard answers. She was at first surprised, as she was herself convinced that promoting mindful awareness and reflection was a suitable approach. She worried that even giving a 'temporary answer' would discourage their thinking and let them rely on her expertise. More importantly, they would return to their habitual way of learning and 'the teacher is the only expert' relationship. Her response was not to give in, but to insist on her teaching method. She encouraged the participants to keep observing their learning progress and comparing our way of learning with their learning habits. One adjustment she made was to offer extra mentoring sessions for some participants who were feeling left far behind. It helped that she understood the participants' perceptions came from their traditional Chinese education, which is almost entirely didactic in nature.

Facing such challenges, you need to reflect by asking yourself why you yourself teach in the way you do. Readers may be reassured that there is no 'standard answer'; everyone works in a different context and in a unique situation, with no one way of doing things. However, it may sometimes mean that you must dig in, as she did. Facing this kind of uncomfortable experience can then help the trainees (and you as trainer too) to learn and discover the essential meanings for yourselves. The process of reflecting on your own response to the demands in applied theatre on teaching and learning is also a promotion of reflection – like a new narrative of education for them and you, learning both in the fictional context and in the context of the setting.

Throughout her course, Yi-Man could not be sure whether these sessions were of benefit to the learners or whether it was just her own rigid and stubborn insistence. So far as she could ascertain, most, possibly all, of the participants showed increased reflectiveness by the end of the training course or later, after the workshop – though, of course, not everyone at the same pace of learning. By the end of the workshop, the students affirmed her insistence and appreciated this way of teaching and learning. She knew that any choice would be taking a risk, and she could not guarantee a positive result. Her pedagogical choices did not come from a vacuum but from her trust in and understanding of applied theatre practice, combined with her own ongoing learning experience and reflection. The same battles and doubts will face you, and you can only hope that your overall demeanour of supportiveness will achieve the same results for your trainees.

At the end of any training course a few participants will still find it hard to reflect critically. But they will observe and appreciate that this way of teaching and learning does bring benefit to the other participants, though they may not be able to identify it so obviously for themselves.

Key factors that support or inhibit training

You must take into account the following central factors that either support or inhibit the learners' management of applied theatre.

Individual experience

We have shown that learners' responses are powerfully influenced by their level of prior experience in applied theatre. This may seem obvious, but too often we still see training based on 'one-size-fits-all' program planning. The adult learners' prior knowledge, skills, and techniques equip them with different frames of reference to assist and at times inhibit their learning. So, they will require different kinds of help to enrich their capacity building. Beginners in applied theatre need a quite different kind of scaffolding from participants with more prior experience. They need to build confidence in the learning methods of applied theatre by accumulating embodied experience and knowledge in the learning process. Participants with a little or some prior applied theatre experience need to take time and practice to strengthen both their capacities to learn and their frames of reference in applied theatre. Therefore, you must take into account and scaffold at least some of their learning based on their particular stage of growth.

Cultural tradition

This relates directly to the point above. It is essential to recognising among the cultural differences and diversity that the learners bring, they may not have had access to much capacity to learn through inquiry-based, dialogical, reflective approaches, which are at the basis of applied theatre, so this poses a challenge to them. The habitual ways of learning in every culture shapes differently the members' perceptions and expectations of learning. If learners hold a traditional – and especially a passive – view of learning, then they may be uncomfortable to take responsibility for their learning. That will inhibit it from the beginning, so this is something you must help them get over, and build into your training program, or you won't get very far.

Teaching how to learn

Yi-Man's study also reinforces how important it is for you to continuously emphasise to the learners their capacity to learn. Applied theatre by its nature can provide the scaffolding that supports this meta-learning. If you pay close attention to enriching the learners' ability to learn – in other words, their generic skills – by structuring your learning content and processes directly to build confidence, this will be a major factor in building their capacity in those skills. They will become more independent and self-constructive learners in applied theatre too.

Reference

Wright, D. (2005). Reflecting on the body in drama education. *Applied Theatre Researcher*, 6/10. Retrieved from: https://www.intellectbooks.com/asset/807/atr-6.10-wright.pdf

9   A deep dive into how adults learn

Preamble

Before we venture to give any more tips and advice, for the sake of any applied theatre learners that we hope you, the readers, can enlighten, we should review what we know about how adults learn – not just from the perspectives of applied theatre makers. We need to put their responses into a coherent pattern of theory and practice to give us confidence that any advice we give you and you give them will be worthwhile, and lead to the deep understanding necessary in applied theatre work.

In Chapters 5–7, we shared and analysed Yi-Man's participants' responses and identified various kinds of knowledge that the training workshop generated for them. This chapter endeavours to explain how and why those participants learnt what they learnt, by elaborating the ways in which knowledge is located within the whole applied theatre experience, as well as the relationships among different kinds of learning that will assist in building capacity. This experience informs our understanding of the stages of growth for any learners in human services professions, which – by definition – deal with serving the needs of complex and unpredictable humans.

The place of knowledge in applied theatre training

Going back to the literature on adult experiential learning, the three knowledge paradigms we mentioned in Chapter 2 identify different 'places of knowledge' in the learning process. The *constructivist* perspective sees learning taken place in the series of conscious mental reflective activities during and/or after attending an experience. In the process of practice and being in the culture of practice, learners develop understanding and skills of knowing through the learning curriculum that evolves out of participation. These theorists tend to emphasise the practical 'know-how' knowledge. *Situated* theorists focus on the socially interactive dimension of learning, perceiving learning as the process of co-participation in the context, not just in the heads of individuals. The *embodied* perspective reminds us of the importance of the learner's body as a primary site of learning. Feeling, doing, and thinking cannot be separated, and operate

DOI: 10.4324/9781003426387-12

together. The sensory, emotional, and affective dimensions in human experience embed the powerful tacit nature of the embodied knowledge.

Each of the three adult experiential learning perspectives puts a different focus on locating the place of learning. However, they cannot ignore the existence of each other. Although learning experience is highly situated, reflection is a necessary tool to articulate what knowledge has been learnt. In a spirit of unification, David Beckett (2004) proposes that bearing reflective questions in mind is a way of effective organic learning. The inferential understanding of 'knowing why' – understanding the reason for action – can develop a more profound knowledge for practice. Beckett also acknowledges the learner's embodiment in the situated context (2001). A holistic learner has regard not only for the cognitive learning but also for social, affective, and physical understanding. Similarly, the embodied learning theorists also do not reject the role of reflection in the learning process but rather bring us back to the central point about human nature: that learning is not a mind–body split.

Throughout this study, we have identified two main domains of necessary knowledge for these learners (applied theatre and generic). Applied theatre knowledge includes concepts, techniques, skills, rationale, and pedagogy as they are articulated by the learners. In varying degrees, learners need to generalise what they learn from the training workshop through reflecting on the embodied experience they go through and observe, just as the constructivists' paradigm proposes. They should be able to state the applied theatre knowledge concretely, although learners at different levels – in our nomenclature, different 'categories' – will conceptualise different levels of depth of knowledge. In contrast, the learners generally should not be expected to articulate their generic learning so well. The way they recognise this aspect of learning will be more based on what they notice about their thinking processes, and their attitudinal and behavioural change during and/or after the training program. The learning evolves through them being in the situation as well as participating in the community of practice. These two aspects of learning will probably have been acquired and identified in different places during the workshop learning process.

There is no one existing adult experiential learning model that can fully make sense of the learning in any applied theatre program. A single domain of adult experiential learning is only valid to inform part of the applied theatre learning experience. The place of knowledge in applied theatre training is the integration of the cognitive, the social, and the embodied learning. The cognitive knowledge about applied theatre must be built up within the social and embodied learning process, in which generic knowledge is generated accordingly.

Aesthetic learning

No matter whether the knowledge is generated through the reflective process or emerges in participation and practice, these certainly do not exist in isolation but are rooted in applied theatre as a kind of aesthetic learning in itself.

Janinka Greenwood (2011) mentions three interrelated aspects of the aesthetic and learning:

- learning about the aesthetic,
- learning through aesthetic experience, and
- visceral, emotional, and intuitive learning, that is not predominantly intellectual but that is located in the body.

Applied theatre learning experience does link those three things together. To apply this idea, we can say a training program is a place: learning *about* applied theatre is *through* specialised experience *not predominantly intellectual* but located in the body. Trainees come to this place to learn about how to use applied theatre, based on their vivid experience which embeds both intellectual and embodied knowing.

Experience generated throughout the training involves multiple ways of knowing/learning, which are akin to John Heron's extended epistemology (1992 – see also Chapter 2). This we will use throughout this chapter to make some kind of sense of the extraordinarily complex organic cognitive, sensory, emotional, and aesthetic tangle, which is how people learn about and within a practical applied theatre program.

According to Heron's theory of personhood, four modes of the psyche (affective, imaginal, conceptual, and practical) are integrated in different combinations, creating four distinct world-views. Each world-view generates one particular form of knowledge (i.e. *experiential, presentational, propositional,* and *practical*). A whole-person holistic learning approach should include these four interrelated ways of knowing. Like other experiential learning models that we have discussed, Heron's theory also tends towards a limited focus on the individual learner's experience, although he does not ignore the learner's interaction with other people. We still find that his identification of four ways of knowing as an epistemic frame is useful to make sense of the learning experience. Prompted by Heron's theory, we acknowledge that no one kind of knowing is sufficient in and of itself to lead to complete understanding about the applied theatre learning experience. Different ways of knowing build on each other to help learners. Knowing is not merely validated through thought and/ or reflection; nor is it only generated through practice in a community. Heron emphasises the equal importance of knowing through full-bodied engagement, located in feeling and emotion, intuition, and imagery. We can apply Heron's four ways of knowing to the planning and experience of applied theatre trainees, alongside the key concepts from the applied theatre literature.

As explained in the earlier chapter, these four kinds of knowing are interwoven, connected with and grounded on each other, instead of being a clear-cut experience on its own. Figure 9.1 illustrates the relationships of applied theatre learning to generic learning, which provide possibilities for each kind of knowing/learning to generate a **specific** kind of capacity to learn, which immediately contributes to the **generic** learning. The capacities to learn strengthen the

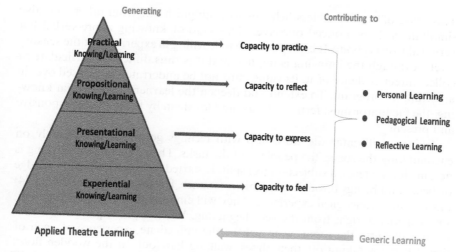

Figure 9.1 Holistic learning model (after Heron 1992).

learner's generic learning to support them, moving onto the next stage of growth in applied theatre learning itself. Those three kinds of generic learning also build the learner's personal and professional agency for supporting their practice and further learning.

Experiential knowing

As Heron stressed, experiential knowing is the bedrock of the other three kinds of knowing. Feeling in experience is not just a resource for learning but also a valid kind of knowing by itself, grounded in the experiential presence of a person in the world and operated by the affective mode of the psyche. It is the state of being in felt-encounter. This is the very foundation of the capacity for feeling.

> Experiential knowing is feeling engaged with what there is, participating, through the perceptual process, in the shared presence of mutual encounter.
>
> (Heron & Reason 2008)

Heron emphasises the experience as not merely individual functioning but also participatory. Knowing is taking place through being present with others in the environment.

> To experience anything is to participate in it, and to participate is both to mould and to encounter, hence experiential reality is always subjective-objective, relative both to the knower and to what is known.
>
> (2008: 2–3)

This sense of connectedness helps us to distinguish self from other, and also simultaneously be noticed ourselves. This kind of knowing is pre-verbal but very real to everybody. It is the entrance to learning **in** experience at the sensory level. Although the knowing is implicit and it is thus difficult to articulate or collect direct evidence of it, its value must not be underrated or glossed over in any training program. To extend and deepen the learners' experiential knowing, the facilitator must fertilise the ground for them by being open, responsive and present.

Trainees will enter the workshop with feelings generated immediately on encountering the space, the people, and the tasks. Their experiential learning is not, in Heron's term, a subject–object split. It started from 'acquiring knowledge of being and beings through empathic resonance, felt participation' (1992: 224) through the pedagogical experience. They will embody this through subtle sensory experience right from the very beginning. When a participant in the program walks into the room, what will be the immediate experience of each of them? Perhaps taking off their shoes, walking barefoot on the wooden floor; seeing a big circle in an open space surrounded by chairs; choosing one of the seats; and sitting down next to somebody. Someone in the circle may feel nervous; someone else may feel enthusiastic; someone else may feel both. Novice learners will feel tense, whereas more experienced learners will feel at home in the familiar setting.

Embodied pedagogy

Embodied pedagogy provides the power for learning, which emphasises participation and dialogue in the social learning process. Body as the primary site of knowing in applied theatre is not based on a grasp of intellectual concepts; rather, it is rooted in experiential knowing. In an effective training program, the participants' experience will be first and foremost through sensing (consciously or unconsciously) their own physicality and their relationship with others. They need to immerse themselves in the embodied learning experience, whether sitting in a big circle, working independently, or in the many smaller group activities that usually characterise applied theatre training sessions. They will listen and be listened to; interact with different people; touch and be touched by others. They will act in the open space, seeing and being seen. Everybody will share the presence of mutual encounter in the room from moment to moment, tacitly and automatically. Gradually, 'a sense of preconceptual communion' (Heron, ibid.: 369) will develop in their shared world within the training workshop. This kind of knowing is the deepened state of awareness that is ingrained in the body.

Feeling and sensitivity to the physical messages and resonances are central to the applied theatre experience. Boal's system of theatre of the oppressed puts it as the priority. For him, it is critical to activate the senses in order to liberate the oppressed body. He proposes his system of exercises and games (2002) to develop people's embodied consciousness 'to feel', 'to listen', and 'to see'. His theory and practice were the foundation of Phase One in Yi-Man's workshop. The participants went through the series of activities (e.g. mirror, image, and sculpture exercises) to extend their awareness of their experiential knowing. They entered into the physical experience and then at the same time they were reminded to focus on sensing their inner feelings and themselves in the space while interacting with others.

Heron reminds us that to lay the groundwork for enhancing experiential knowing, those emotional elements of confidence, attunement, felt resonance, and positive arousal are also critical to support effective learning. The facilitator should work towards 'eliciting a positive emotional attitude within the learner' and help 'learners generate and sustain emotional arousal among themselves'.

> People learn more effectively when they are enjoying themselves and what they are doing; when they are satisfying some felt need or interest and are emotionally involved in what has personal relevance to them; when they feel good about the whole idea of learning and the exercise of their learning competence; when they feel confident, secure and in a low threat, cooperative, non-competitive situation.
>
> (1992: 229)

A healthy social space – building a positive relationship with trust and a sense of supportive community – is the key to a successful entry into drama. It is the basis of any kind of applied theatre learning in the aesthetic space. Therefore, where participants are isolated, and the emotional relationship among them falls apart, this poor social connectedness will make it impossible for fully effective learning to happen. Normally, participants will bring a high level of interest or at least curiosity to applied theatre training. In Yi-Man's first interview before her workshop started, they described positive past experiences and expectations; both beginners and experienced learners felt excited to be in touch with applied theatre. A positive emotional attitude to applied theatre must therefore be generated right from the beginning by the training program and then supported by the growing pedagogical experience which should sustain and – in most cases – increase the trainees' emotional arousal and willingness to try throughout the process. For Yi-Man, a few Category One participants felt confused and lost in the process at some points, but it did not diminish their interest in being in the training workshop nor their confidence in applied theatre. Her intention as facilitator was from the start to make all efforts to build an inclusive, caring, encouraging atmosphere to allow participants to feel safe and comfortable both in connecting with others and in looking into their inner selves.

The pedagogical experience initiated through the design of the training program will thus act like an undercurrent to irrigate the soil for experiential knowing. The learning for the participants will emerge at the experiential level first through their immediate sensory memory, which, as we have demonstrated earlier, significantly contributes to their later understanding of applied theatre.

In applied theatre learning, experiential knowing is generated not only in the real-life social context but also in the drama/applied theatre exercises and fictional dramatic contexts. It is a truism of drama education that emotion is at the heart of the drama experience. More than just seeking or building a positive atmosphere or culture for learners to feel safe and relaxed, the facilitator or teacher will use emotions (not always positive but always authentic) for deepening the learning. As discussed in detail in Chapter 2, the relationship of the emotions to drama has been an important theme of research in drama education. David Wright makes explicit the relationship between drama and feeling.

> Drama education, in contrast to other forms of education not in or of the arts, is a field of feeling – and needs to be taught as a field of feeling – as much as it is a field of knowing. Without feeling, drama is of little consequence. The sensitive nature of the excursion into feeling is a necessary part of the learning in drama.
>
> (Wright, 2005: page unnumbered)

No matter whether doing exercises and activities in the theatre of the oppressed, working in role in process drama, or performing in participatory theatre, or doing other applied theatre activities preferred by the facilitator, good applied theatre practice is always conscious of the power of using the affective domain to heighten the learning experience. Playing in role in drama purposefully engages the participants' emotions within a 'no penalty zone' to facilitate deep learning. In the imagined world, under the protection of role the learner steps into the world of otherness and feels as those others, either positively or negatively. Something as simple as embodying images for a character or personal situation in an exercise, or just watching others' performances, will also strike us with these emotions. Learning can be taking place through the interaction between feelings in personal real-world experience and the feelings evoked by the dramatic world.

Bolton calls feeling and emotion created in drama the 'second order experience'. This experience creates distance for the learner to review and examine the meaning of life. He explains,

> In drama we require a heightened awareness of the interaction of two worlds, not an avoidance of the fictitious so that nothing is felt, nor an escape into the fictitious so that everything is felt but nothing is understood. The emotion that is experienced then is really a compound of emotions that is prompted by both the contexts.
>
> (1986: 106)

The affective experience in applied theatre that encourages participants to enter into another's viewpoint is the essence of the empathic understanding that is promoted in experiential learning. Applied theatre not only exteriorises internal domains of feeling about other participants and self in the empathic face-to-face relationships. It also provides the opportunity for the participants to build empathy by exploring their wider human social relations through emotional learning. This resonates with the commentaries of Yi-Man's participants who identified with the impact of the feelings the characters felt when they embodied themselves in the images of the oppressed, the stories of process dramas and when playing the protagonists in the participatory theatre performance.

To summarise, experiential knowing/learning in any human services field is cultivated in both real and fictional contexts. In the real social context, the whole-person knowing of self and others is enriched through developing participants' sensitivity and mindful awareness to notice various felt-encounters constantly in process. As well as creating a culture that honours feeling as a way of knowing and a positive influence on the learning process, the *capacity to feel* is nurtured in at the foundational level through rich experiential knowing.

Presentational knowing

This kind of knowing is processed through an intuitive grasp of the imaginal patterns expressed in various art forms. The learning experience through this way of knowing directly informs experiential knowing/learning and is also informed by it. Expressive activities bring the unconscious and unarticulated experiential knowing into a communicative form open to reflection. This can be recognised itself as a kind of knowledge, and because drama is a group art form it provides a platform for individuals to connect with each other in the learning space, to provide them with a bridge between experiential and propositional knowing.

In Heron's view, art manifests the tacit knowledge and emotional experience inherent in images through shape, sound, movement, metaphor and symbol in order to reveal the underlying pattern of things. He validates that by borrowing ideas from theories of expression and the work of Susanne Langer (see Chapter 2). Art as symbol of feeling makes the affective dimension of knowledge explicit.

Applied theatre's use of aesthetic patterns like symbols and signs, spaces, images, metaphors, stories, movements, are all main components of a presentational way of knowing. Chris Seeley identifies four relevant elements in her extended epistemology of presentational knowing – which is also aligned with the applied theatre learning process. They are:

i. **Sensuous encountering**: using all our ways of sensing to experience the world directly with a whole-body sense of curiosity and appreciation for the glorious mundane;
ii. **Suspending**: hanging fire with fresh rounds of clever intellectual retorts in order to become more deeply acquainted with the responses to experience of our more-than-brainy bodies to the more-than-human world;

iii. **Bodying-forth**: inviting imaginative impulses to express themselves through the media of our bodies without our intellects throwing a spanner in the works and crushing those responses with misplaced rationality or premature editing and critique;
iv. **Being in-formed**: becoming beings whose living and actions form and are informed by the rich experiences, surprises, provocations and evocations of presentational knowing, both as perceivers and as creators.

(Seeley & Reason, 2008: 30–31)

These four elements do not have a separate existence and each state offers something to the others. They co-arise, and in time they blur into one another. As we have shown just above, feeling via the senses is the foundation for all ways of knowing. Particularly in applied theatre, it is important for participants to open up, as well as to sharpen their capacity to feel, in order to learn effectively in the process.

Sensuous encountering is also the starting base for presentational knowing in most genres of applied theatre. Learning through the presentational way of knowing, participants in applied theatre are asked to temporarily turn off their intellect (a paradox that will be explained below). They suspend their disbelief to step into the aesthetic space to explore new meaning from the unknown that lies beyond reality's usual images and knowledge. Echoing Langer, the experience in the art intends to create 'strangeness, separateness, other-ness' for insightful learning. To do this, participants have to delay their judgement and the analysis of meaning and allow their expressive knowing to bring them a new way of seeing. Let us take a simple example from Phase One in Yi-Man's workshop. In the sculpting exercise, participants in pairs were asked to create a series of free-form images by using their partner's body. Instead of planning ahead, they were encouraged to just follow their immediate feeling and make different human statues so that they could see what they had created and be surprised by it. Participants had to apply the same spirit to working within the dramatic context to submerge themselves into the life of the story and the characters' journey. Suspending the intellect does not mean 'not thinking' but highlighting the process of 'not-knowing'. In the applied theatre learning experience, the element of suspension is of considerable importance within the presentational way of knowing. The habitual and dominant cognitive mind is placed into the background for a while, to give space where the affective mind can become both engaged and then visible.

While coming to know through sensuous encountering and suspending, bodying-forth becomes the yield of both. Seeley and Reason (2008) explains,

...communicative meaning is first incarnate in the gestures by which the body spontaneously expresses feeling and responds to change in its affective environment.

The gesture is spontaneous and immediate. It is not an arbitrary sign that we mentally attach to a particular emotion or feeling; rather, the gesture is the bodying-forth of that emotion into the world, it is that feeling of delight or of anguish in its tangible, visible aspect.

(ibid. 2008: 40)

Since body is the basic means of mediation in applied theatre practice, learners allow the presentational knowing through the body to be mediated by different kinds of materials used for expression. When participants in applied theatre work with the body within different frames of the exercises and activities, they make spontaneous physical expressions that represent their existing understanding and interpretation by using their body, and they also respond to others' bodies. They can be encouraged to try out different ways to use their body and collective bodies through free kinaesthetic imagination, creatively and actively. The genre will provide a new physical experience for most learners to elicit their new/unconscious understanding of the self, others, and the environment. This direct experience intentionally builds a platform for them to observe and reflect through their embodied awareness during the practice. Their heightened awareness of the emotion and action in this process raises thoughts and ideas for participants' further thinking. Usage of embodied experience in applied theatre widens learners' imaginations, which are not limited to the real context, but are also working in the fictional context.

The presentational way of knowing can also be rooted in the playing of roles in drama. Role-playing in applied theatre expands the bodylines of social relations to include words. For trainees, by engaging in a physical gesture or non-verbal language to accompany their act of communicative expression, at the same time they are representing the life of the characters they play. The body becomes a metaphor. Through a series of non-scripted collaborative and improvised enactments, players employ the characters' language and step into those others' emotional status, to learn about their lives and situations. Through the range of performance forms offered in applied theatre, trainees can examine the lives of the others in action, neither merely in mental activity nor just sharing verbally. In order to communicate, they first search for an appropriate expressive form to create the performance. Bodying-forth is irreplaceable in the applied theatre process. Participants can never plan exactly or expect a particular outcome of their explorations. Applied theatre as the way of knowing/learning is always provisional and in the process of becoming. It is highly experimental by nature.

'Being in-formed' will emerge from going through the above three elements (i.e. sensuous encountering, suspending, and bodying-forth). A new way of seeing is generated through imagination and intuition in the expressive knowing process. It is a foundation for new thoughts, ideas, and behaviour – a new self-awareness. In applied theatre, mindful awareness is aroused for informing learning through sensuous encountering, suspending judgement and disbelief and allowing the body to work in spontaneous flow. Participants perceive through experiential knowing and create through presentational knowing. The human ability to hold dual reality in mind is one of the primary drivers of learning in drama process, as Gavin Bolton (1984: 153) explained in Chapter 3. Participants see themselves act while acting; and observe themselves in action and reflect on it. Their existing world-views and understandings can be noticed and visualised, which makes them accessible for use in dialogue with others. During this process, new meaning is created and codified to bring insight to learners.

Working in applied theatre, trainees invoke the presentational way of knowing by using various expressive forms to communicate the experience of experiential knowing or to generate expressive knowledge by itself from the exercises and activities. While they work in the forms, they are also acquiring skills to use the forms and practise them through embodiment. This is congruent with what Boal says about the human body,

> ...to control the means of theatrical production man must first of all control his own body, know his own body, in order to be capable of making it more expressive.
>
> (1979: 124–125)

To learn to be more expressive, they are also required to develop the sensitivity to raise conscious awareness in the process. By embodying through applied theatre, participants are also invited to constantly connect their outside worlds into the mental and emotional place that leads them to be open to learning as whole-person learners. Participants working in various forms of applied theatre prepare themselves to be familiar with using and controlling their body to learn how to create, respond, and communicate. As the confidence of mastering the forms increases, their *capacity to express* will also flourish vividly through this way of knowing/learning.

Propositional knowing

This way of knowing is the traditional kind of knowledge based on cognitive ideas, concepts, and words. It is the 'knowledge-about' that is expressed in propositions – 'statements which use language to assert facts about the world, laws that make generalizations about facts and theories that organize the laws' (Heron & Reason, 2008: 373–374). Heron emphasises that propositional knowing should be coherent and consistent with presentational and experiential knowing. It is not a type of knowing that is split off as a conceptualised entity and privileged above those, as in many conventional educational assumptions. It is the knowing which Heron calls 'subject–object transaction' that 'you need to go deeper into the subject in order to go deeper into the object, that is, if you want to get into the object' (1992: 170). To go deeper into the object through the subject, we go through the process of being present and opening ourselves to participation in and with it, along with the flow of exercising imagination within perception. This way of knowing will then reveal what had been disclosed by expressing the conceptualising object and naming it as a proposition.

In learning applied theatre, the knowledge-about is usually constructed by learners' own reflection. The role of reflection is the catalyst for the propositional knowledge. Using Heron's notion, through experiential knowing in the encounter, presence generates *feeling*; presentational knowing brings feeling into *consciousness* which, in the conceptual mode for theorising the learning, becomes food for *reflection*.

Propositional knowing through reflection can be set up for trainees through various kinds of tasks, in verbal and written formats, individually and collectively. They can come to learn more generically about 'what is applied theatre' and 'how it works'. There will be a number of common reflective spaces which can serve this purpose within a workshop or program. Common general reflective spaces include whole-group discussions, at the end and/or the opening of each session; during a course-ending reflective discussion; and, of course, writing an individual reflective journal. These places for reflection are different, but they serve similar functions. In these propositional learning spaces, participants are encouraged to use their reflective conscious awareness to make sense of the embodied experience. They turn on cognitive analysis to conceptualise 'what is applied theatre' and 'how it works' through critical discourse and critical reflection. Public and open collective discussion is a significant means for trainees to tap into their own observations and discoveries in the process and begin to share with others the meanings that they have implicitly understood in the experience. Personal critical reflection can be shared publicly to articulate what's in the trainees' minds and also serve as a generated wisdom to pass on to help others' – and their own – further reflection.

Knowledge about applied theatre is a kind of self-constructive propositional knowing. It is crucial for learners to have their own private reflective space for contemplation. Writing or dictating a reflective journal we think is one of the best platforms for this space. Going through their personal experiences and the active dialogues with others, learners will organise and document their own meaning and construct their own theory of applied theatre as far as they are able at each stage. Reflective ability is vital but cannot be taken for granted. Full and wholehearted participation in the whole program is essential. With that, the applied theatre itself is a generative space for reflection with opportunities for learners to practise using cognitive thinking to actively observe and analyse what is happening in the moment. It is possible to train learners to reflect more deeply. We may speculate that in all probability, this will enhance their overall quality of reflection.

Practical knowing

Practical knowing is 'knowing how-to-do, how to engage in, some class of action or practice' (Heron & Reason, 2008: 375). It emerges from the experiential to the presentational to the propositional. Although it is immediately grounded in propositional knowing, it has to go beyond the descriptive concepts into the autonomous competence whereby learners can show they are able to use their skills. In learning how to practise applied theatre, practitioners need to have knowledge-how, tacit knowledge, and the ability to perform, in order to use practical knowledge effectively. Peter Jarvis (1994) stresses that 'knowing how' and 'being able' are not synonymous. Practical knowledge includes two inter-related dimensions other than the ability to do something: knowledge-how and tacit knowledge. They are both embodied in the individual who performs the practice.

Jarvis analyses six factors in the getting of practical knowledge: learning knowledge-how; learning how in practice; acquiring tacit knowledge by forgetting; acquiring tacit knowledge by learning pre-consciously; acquiring knowledge-how by reflective learning; and continuing learning and education that relates theory to practice (1994: 39–42). In addition to Heron's theory, it is helpful to take Jarvis's ideas to elaborate where the practical way of knowing is located in applied theatre training. For learning knowledge-how, Jarvis suggests that we can acquire it by four different processes, learning through:

- taught instructions (e.g. lectures and demonstrations)
- practice (going through stages of observing, trying-out, and independent practice)
- reflective learning (turning the discovery from action into a new body of practical knowledge)
- continuous learning and education.

Instructions

We will focus on the first three of those processes, although continuity of learning is crucial to the ongoing career of the applied theatre practitioner or human services worker – that goes without saying. In training, learning knowledge-how (know-how) through instructions and in practice should always come together. Whatever kind of applied theatre is required, trainees need learnt know-how to practise, of course. This will begin with the trainer's introduction, instruction, or demonstration – at least briefly to describe how the practice functions and its preliminary procedures, if necessary, by giving a demonstration. Then, the learners will spend most of their time learning from their own embodiment of the work individually or collectively. In the early parts of the program, the learners will engage in the practice mainly as participants; later, it will gradually shift to engage them as facilitators. Learning know-how as participants will come about for them mainly through embodying the steps and sequences of the exercises, activities, and dramas. As they become more confident in these practices, know-how as facilitators needs to be cultivated through the learners leading the work independently in activities like micro-teaching or, if possible, dramatic internships or placements, where they will learn to exercise their planning and facilitation skills.

Practice

As propositional know-how is performed in practice, then new observations and discoveries as well as new skills in ongoing activities will feed in to enrich the new know-how. Moreover, as Jarvis mentions, tacit knowledge can be acquired by forgetting and pre-conscious learning. As the participants gain in expertise during the practical work, they tend to forget the existence of the original rules – which still remain in play at a low consciousness level. The knowledge is gradually internalised and accumulated without conscious awareness. By the natural process of working through direct experience, humans learn pre-consciously from their embodied social practice within the learning community; the tacit dimension of practical knowledge – which is impossible to articulate – develops within the individuals and the group. Through participation and facilitation, their minds and bodies commit the skills to memory.

The *capacity to practise* is basically embedded in all capacities generated in the process of the other three ways of knowing. It is directed by *propositional* learning, inspired by *presentational* forms, and rooted in and continually refreshed by *experiential* encounters. So we can say the capacity to practise includes the capacity to feel, to express, and to reflect. Learners move from learning basic skills (like making an image or a group freeze-frame by using the body) to practising more complex and integrated and more dramatic genres at later stages – extending the basic exercises into dramatic narratives with new conventions, for which more and more they become responsible for devising the structures and stratagems. This new capacity to create drama for themselves needs to find an outlet, first in mature processes and performance among the group. Then, ideally, they need to find real purposes to devise stratagems for outsiders, where they must put their money where their mouth is. However, it is still crucial to include this phase within the training program itself, not just to cast the learners out on the stream, because when they hit the unpredictability of real clients and consumers, they will inevitably discover the great ideas they planned in the program classes will not work as expected, but they will still have the facilitator's and their group's support to help them reflect, find out why…and, if necessary, restore their morale…

Reflection

…And this, of course, is where reflection becomes a very real part of practical knowing, among the most essential capacities for the applied theatre practitioner, who will rarely be presented with a safe and predictable environment, or a support system to rely on.

The planning and facilitation skills that the learners have been acquiring, conscious and tacit, will – by this latter stage – have also included a lot of preliminary reflection, and learning how to reflect on the exercise and dramatic activities. These have throughout, until now, been carried out in the penalty-free zone of the classroom, as participants gradually engage in learning to participate in more and more complex dramas, then to stretch their wings in taking on the beginnings of facilitating within and among the group. With various opportunities for practice, the participants also will have the ability to cooperate with others, including difficult or resistant others, which is also one of the main ingredients of the capacity to practise. Not least, the concepts and pedagogy gained along with the implicit knowledge thus become part of the critical source of capacity building through the practical way of knowing. Learning experiences in the applied theatre program will, in fact, have included multiple ways of knowing. Each way of learning how to know, and what kinds of knowing matter in which situation, specifically nurtures its own distinct capacity. To reiterate, all ways of knowing and the capacities they generate cross-fertilise each other, and sometimes this occurs simultaneously. It is a dynamic interplay among the activities, mediated by an intuitive grasp of imaginal patterns in the practice, and then naming propositionally the quality that has been identified as creating the learning.

Segue

This chapter has been perhaps unexpectedly theoretical, as we come to grips with what it means to learn (anything). In the final chapter, we will bring the discussion home to show how all these ways of learning can inform our understanding of the four aspects of learning that have been identified in this book (i.e.: applied theatre learning, personal learning, pedagogical learning, and reflective learning). We can then start to look at our learners, at whatever stage they are, and work out their needs. This is the essential beginning of applied theatre program planning.

References

Beckett, D. (2001). Ontological performance: Bodies, identities and learning. *Studies in the Education of Adults, 33*(1), 35–48.

Beckett, D. (2004). Embodied competence and generic skill: The emergence of inferential understanding. *Educational Philosophy and Theory, 36*(5), 497–508.

Boal, A. (1979). *Theatre of the oppressed*. London: Pluto Press.

Boal, A. (2002). *Games for actors and non-actors* (2nd Ed.). London: Routledge.

Bolton, G. (1984). *Drama as education*. London: Longman.

Bolton, G. (1986). Emotion in the dramatic process: Is it an adjective or a verb? In D. Davis & C. Lawrence (Eds.), *Gavin Bolton: Selected writings* (pp. 100–107). London: Longman.

Greenwood, J. (2011). Aesthetic learning, and learning through the aesthetic. In S. Schonmann (Ed.), *Key concepts in theatre/drama education* (pp. 47–52). Rotterdam: Sense.

Heron, J. (1992). *Feeling and personhood: Psychology in another key*. London: Sage.

Heron, J., & Reason, P. (2008). Extending epistemology within a co-operative inquiry. In P. Reason & H. Bradbury (Eds.), *The SAGE handbook of action research: Participative inquiry and practice* (2nd ed., pp. 366–380). London: SAGE.

Jarvis, P. (1994). Learning practical knowledge. *Journal of Further and Higher Education Research and Development, 18*(1), 31–43.

Seeley, C., & Reason, P. (2008). Expressions of energy: An epistemology of presentational knowing. In P. Liamputtong & J. Rumbold (Eds.), *Knowing differently: Arts-based & collaborative research methods* (pp. 25–46). New York: Nova Science.

Wright, D. (2005). Reflecting on the body in drama education. *Applied Theatre Researcher, 6/10*. Retrieved from: https://www.intellectbooks.com/asset/807/atr-6.10-wright.pdf

10   Applied theatre without tears

Sorting the sheep from the goats

Yi-Man's deep and thorough study clearly showed that learners' responses to an applied theatre training program are powerfully influenced by their level of prior experience in applied theatre. One might (and we will) generalise out from this to suggest this is true of nearly all adult training programs in human services which include participants with different ages, experiences, and cultural backgrounds. Their prior knowledge, skills, and techniques equip the participants with different frames of reference assisting or at times inhibiting their learning in the process. Therefore, participants with different levels of experience will require different kinds of help to enrich their capacity building process.

At the outset, Yi-Man, not quite arbitrarily, but based on instinct and what she saw from the participants, decided to use a three-level categorisation of previous applied theatre experience: beginners, those with a basic familiarity of some kind, and more experienced. This turned out to be revealing, trustworthy, and helpful, and has provided us with much of Part II, particularly the chapter on applied theatre itself (Chapter 5). So, as the base level of our advice here, we will revisit that same categorisation. This is bound to be one of the major considerations for trainers and facilitators to take account of and remain cognisant of throughout the whole program. One size will not fit all.

Prior professional records, histories, or credentials are a place to start – though these can, of course, be quite misleading unless they are well-contextualised and you are well-informed. Then, careful pre-training consultation and backgrounding of your client learners, of the sort that Yi-Man did, with correspondence, instructions, and interviews, is ideal. However, you might find yourself dealing with a scratch group of whose provenance you have little idea. If so, the early part of your program needs to be largely diagnostic, ascertaining the learners' levels of skills, experience, and savvy (knowing-how, as Jarvis more properly calls it [1994]), both formal and informal. This will happen quite naturally through the practical work that is likely to form the first part of your program, so long as this is set up to be engaging to all, busy, and with varied levels of challenge. Differences of capacity, confidence, and experience will all reveal

DOI: 10.4324/9781003426387-13

themselves to the eagle-eyed facilitator, which is what you must be! Make sure that from the start you have some kind of recording device or checklist that can identify those differences as they appear in all the individuals. You may be luckier than Yi-Man and be working with a colleague, assistant, or outside observer, in which case each session must be followed by a diagnostic debriefing on what you both observed.

Beginners in applied theatre need a quite different kind of scaffolding from participants with some prior experience. They need to build confidence in the teaching and learning methods of applied theatre by accumulating embodied experience and knowledge within the learning process. Participants with a little prior applied theatre experience need to take time and practice to strengthen both their capacities to learn and their frames of reference in applied theatre. By increasing their applied theatre experience, the capacities to learn generated in the process will enrich the participants' efficacy in learning. Participants who have more substantial experience can be expected to be more critical, and better able to understand what underlies the training, to be more focused on you, the facilitator, and to be more ready to apply the activities to their own settings. Therefore, any facilitator must take into account and scaffold the participants' learning based on their particular stage of growth.

In order to gain more understanding of the impact of prior experience in the participants' learning process we can cross-reference this tripartite categorisation to explore those differences with three further criteria, which will then assist our future planning: *emotional response, reaction to new learning*, and *applying their learning*.

Emotional response

The first criterion relates to the contrasting emotional reactions the participants will display when they encounter applied theatre. Category One participants (the beginners), lacking experience, will display the most visible emotional responses to the learning – though this may be expressed in passivity, resistance, or reluctance (easy for the eagle-eyed to spot). They have no background knowledge or experience to support them in what is a new, and for many a strange, learning environment, unlike any they have come across before. They won't know how to bodily participate in the training workshop. Lack of prior experience will probably make them feel anxious as they struggle to enter the new way of learning. Although they will probably be excited, or at least curious, and ready to come for learning, at the same time they will doubt their performance as participants. They will not know what they 'should' do, and they will not easily make sense of the meaning of the activities. Many will probably judge themselves to be 'uncreative' and 'incapable', especially in the earlier phase of learning, and even continue thinking in this way when they encounter difficulties in the later phases.

Category Two participants (those with at least a little experience) will also sometimes feel frustrated and confused. However, they will not assume their confusion and frustration results from being incapable of learning new applied theatre. They will probably quickly turn the emotional responses into an insight for personal learning. They will perceive the program as a process of learning which itself is likely to further motivate their improvement, and they will be able to evaluate how and how much.

Category Three participants will be rather more detached and able to observe their own and others' emotional responses. Learning from their prior experience, they will not be easily disturbed by the emotional fluctuations generated in the learning process. They will manage their immediate emotional reactions to activities in the program and see them as irrelevant to their learning ability.

Reaction to new learning

The second criterion is the participants' responses, in their categories, towards encountering new learning. Category One participants are unlikely to have any previous applied theatre frame of reference, to support and guide their new learning. It is not unlikely that they may come with baggage of their own, in the form of familiarity with more conventional forms of theatre. This may well unsettle them, puzzle and confuse them, as they find what they are doing does not accord with their own prior theatrical experience.

On the whole, they will not understand how the activities are going to work and are likely to think there is a set of rules to which they should conform. They may well be disconcerted by the constantly questioning and negotiating approach of the good facilitator, and the indeterminate nature of many of the activities you set up, and they may want the reassurance of a tighter structure (especially those who are used to more rigid and didactic teaching). Beginners will pose a range of questions, but have very limited ability to proceed towards answers at this stage. They will stay with their emotional response when they feel difficulty in learning new things. In most cases, it will cost them considerable effort to manage the broad disparity between internal knowledge and external new experience.

Category Two participants may be expected to respond differently when they encounter a brand-new experience or kind of applied theatre. They will want to actively discuss, analyse, and make sense of new activities, supported by their previous knowledge and experience, and they will actively find new and deeper learning in the activities they have come across before. They will also pose questions when they do not understand what has happened – but questions at a deeper and more sophisticated level than the mainly procedural questions asked by beginners. They will take unfamiliar experience as the resource to build on their existing understanding in applied theatre. In contrast, most of Category One learners may not initially see building on unfamiliar knowledge as a necessary process of learning; instead, they may attribute the unfamiliarity to their personal inadequacy. The Category Two learners will also show a growing autonomy in the learning process.

Category Three learners may be expected to perform more independently. They will be able to contemplate and create meaning out of new activities and have deeper insights into those activities they have previously taken part in or learnt. They are conscious of making choices about what they want to further develop according to their personal learning objectives, and they will be inspired to assimilate new things into their current knowledge to create new understanding and better practice.

Applying their learning

The third criterion is how they will approach applying the new learning. Category One participants will tend to find their ideas for applying activities by copying and imitating the surface features and steps. Category Two participants will analyse the activities and if they are already involved in professional settings, integrate them into their existing work. They will be able to give reasons for the ways they will use the activities. For the Category Three participants, they will be much more able to make sense of the learning for their own use. They will think about how to do it, and do it differently, to modify the activities for their own needs.

The different approaches to creating applied theatre reflect the participants' conception of their learning as it is rooted in their frames of reference. Learners in any experiential field will bring their own thinking about the learning process to accommodate new experience. Advanced learners who have a broader frame of reference have more choices of possible ways to view the experience. Jennifer Moon (2004: 42) describes our applied theatre learners nicely:

> as a learner becomes more sophisticated in the manner in which she conceives of knowledge, we can say that she becomes more flexible in the manner in which she works with knowledge – and more flexible in the way in which she sees knowledge is used by others.

Beginners tend to see applied theatre knowledge as a kind of received knowledge that they have to memorise and reproduce in order to learn; the more experienced learners get to recognise that the learning is constructed through the internalising process of building the knowledge for themselves. The observable responses of the learners to the applied theatre activities and program can be summarised, as illustrated in Table 10.1.

This diagram can help us to identify the various learning conditions in each stage of learning. The learning conditions are not fixed but fluid and change with increasing experience. Even though for Category One learners those limitations may be apparent at the start, all the learners will be likely to make some progress by the end of the training program. Some learners will make significant journeys towards enablement. In general, the participants with more

Table 10.1 Typical learning responses by category

Category One	Category Two	Category Three
comparatively more emotional blocks; sense of uncertainty in the learning process;	fewer emotional blocks, and treats obstacles not as themselves being incapable to learn but as an insight to personal learning;	relatively free from emotional blocks; emotion is itself a source for learning;
comparatively low learning confidence, self-doubt, low self-efficacy;	more learning confidence;	confident, self-directed;
lack of frame of reference to support the new learning and, still in the process of making sense of 'knowing-that', tends to ask surface and procedural questions;	enough frames of reference to support deeper observation and analysis for understanding the learning;	asks deeper questions; understands that knowing-that and knowing-how leads to more knowing-why knowledge;
knowledge is passively received as beginning learner; copies and imitates the surface features and steps as an entry point to learn for practice	knowledge is constructed; analysis of the activities and integration of the knowledge into their existing work; can take unfamiliar experience as a new resource to build on their existing understanding	knowledge is constructed and provisional; not only studies the new knowledge, but creates/ modifies new meaning for their own use; builds on the new learning with further insight.

experience will be more confident, flexible, reflective, independent, self-directed, and find less emotional disruption in the learning process. The stages of growth of applied theatre learners rely on their levels of learning experience, to equip them with learning frames of reference to enhance their ongoing learning. Those frames of reference provide guidance for the learners to select their focuses of concern, to perceive the process of learning and the nature of knowledge, as well as to give them the capability to learn through participating in the applied theatre activities.

The different stages of learning among the three categories show that applied theatre learning is very much a kind of constructivist knowledge. Learners build on their own knowledge in every applied theatre experience. They grasp new experiences and think about them to construct their understanding of the method. When they get a chance for a revisit through participation and/or practice, they form new insights in comparing with their existing understanding and modify that if necessary. They bring to the surface of their understanding what they have learnt about applied theatre based on reflecting and integrating their observations from the experience to create concepts for making sense of the practice. Going through this mental activity, learners can learn to articulate the knowledge concretely to facilitate their future learning.

Adult trainees select things to learn according to their frames of reference. As we have stressed, there are two central modes of perception (participant and facilitator) in which they operate, creating different focal awareness towards perceiving their learning in the experience. By operating in the participant mode, the learners will tend first to place their personal responses at the centre of the learning process. By operating in the facilitator mode, the learners will put their focus on facilitation, thinking about the methods and rationales of teaching and observing others' learning responses. They will use more objective eyes to see what is happening. Our novices will tend at first just to use participant mode; as they get more experienced they will move more into facilitator mode. Then they will be able to learn at a more advanced level, to be more independent, self-directed, reflexive, and with a critical mind.

Five levels of capacity

Following many years' experience and analysis of applied theatre we have both found that, beyond training, it is useful to broaden out Yi-Man's rough three-step categorisation of the relationship of experience to learning prowess, to look at where everybody involved in applied theatre is in terms of their current capacity, as a prelude to building further capacity and greater expertise. Along with analysis of two other training programs world-wide, we identified a five-level Scale of Capacity. Each level, we found, is readily distinguished by the hurdles between them that practitioners or learners must overcome, to reach the next level.[1]

We named the levels *Readiness, Experience, Adoption, Ownership*, and *Mastery* (Table 10.2).

Table 10.2 Five levels of applied theatre capacity

Level	Hurdle
1. **Readiness**	*Willingness to engage collaboratively*
2. **Experience**	*Confidence to go on, and a little basket of skills*
3. **Adoption**	*Applying the skills*
4. **Ownership**	*Robustness in correction and readiness to lead and change*
5. **Mastery**	

Source : This table indicates the five levels of applied theatre capacity, from complete unfamiliarity to mastery, along with the hurdles necessary to move from one to the next.

Level 1: readiness

The first level is *Readiness*. Even to make a start, a worker or would-be worker in applied theatre must have an openness to experiencing and experimenting, with not only a new art form but also a new pedagogy; a willingness to encounter disruptions to their expectations and familiarity. In many cases, of people with some conventional drama or theatre experience but no understanding of applied theatre, they must be ready to shed some of their assumptions relating to their prior experience and understanding of drama.

1st Hurdle: willingness to engage collaboratively

The first hurdle requirement is an active willingness – keenness – to engage in an ensemble, and readiness to manage and control the emotions and empathy aroused by drama. If you are selecting either trainees or untrained company members, you should make sure that these qualities of readiness are expressly articulated by the applicants. That was at least true for all Yi-Man's study participants, who came by choice and ready to learn. They can't do applied theatre with other people if they are themselves unconvinced of its power.

Level 2: experience

The second level is *Experience*, direct and personal. It is difficult or impossible for would-be applied theatre practitioners to understand fully any form of participatory theatre, appreciate its potency and how it feels, or manage their own clients effectively in those experiences, without having undergone some live dramatic experience. That will give them at least a taste of the particular aesthetic combination of embodied experience, emotional engagement, cognitive reasoning, and reflection.

2nd hurdle: confidence to go on, and a little basket of skills

The hurdle requirement to get beyond this stage is to demonstrate sufficient confidence, and enough understanding of basic skills to begin to extrapolate from the experience and start at least thinking about implementing the next stage themselves.

Alternative classification

Depending on the context of learning or practice, these first two preliminary stages can be – and sometimes need to be – reversed, for learners with ignorance and no motivation, as can often be the case in all sorts of drama workshops. The dramatic *experience* needs to come as a welcome surprise, which generates readiness to learn more. We can think of countless groups of headteachers, judges, police, post office workers, senior administrators, and trainees in a multitude of fields, with whom we have worked, that appear to have no prior connection with theatre. They frequently encounter theatre with scepticism or at least suspicion, fuelled by their own prior life experiences or assumptions of the word. For all of them, the actual pleasurable physical experience is essential to break down their resistance and replace it with *readiness*. Whichever way round these two stages happen, each is entirely dependent on the other. All those who come cold into applied theatre workshops or training programs may start with no knowledge or very limited, but they will experience various enjoyable activities, which change whatever perception of applied theatre they might have had and build a basis of basic techniques and simple skills. This learning will provide them with a Level 1 keenness, willingness, and openness, which together will form a basis for their moving into Level 3.

Level 3: adoption

Levels 1 and 2 learners move from *readiness* and *experience* to *adoption* (Level 3). They will have leapt their hurdle with some basic concepts, the beginnings of confidence in the efficacy of applied theatre and expectations of it, as well as some simple knowledge of applied theatre activities. This is where a training facilitator – or for an untrained company member, a supportive director along with fellow company members – is essential in the first place. This will help to provide the neophyte with a deeper understanding and more practice in their sketchily known concepts, exercises, and activities, and some new techniques and activities which they can understand and build upon those for particular purposes. A mature level of adoption arrives when they can apply within their own practice new structures, strategies, and techniques that they have experienced, and become at least cognisant of the pedagogy or negotiation necessary in their own context. In addition, the practitioner will be gaining a more sophisticated awareness of the skills of their training facilitator or company leaders.

3rd hurdle: applying the skills

The ability to apply what they have learned beyond their training or company environment, together with the confidence to look beyond there, is the next hurdle requirement.

Level 4: ownership

An early characteristic of *ownership* (Level 4) is being able to observe the facilitator's or company leaders' practices and accurately read their thinking. Practitioners at this level have also acquired a bank of knowledge and skills in applied theatre gained from their previous learning experience and practice. They will have acquired the ability to take their bank of structures, strategies, and techniques and apply them in both new and unfamiliar contexts. They will be prepared to start leading company work or facilitating training themselves. This level not only demands increased control of the medium, but the ability to cope with trial and error.

4th hurdle: robustness in correction and readiness to lead and change

The hurdle requirement for this level entails 1. being confident, skilled, and robust enough to reflect on and correct or deal with their own errors and failures, rather than be deterred, defensive, dependent, or demoralised; 2. Being ready to initiate, lead, and change as necessary new applied theatre projects, and deal with the inevitable slings and arrows!

Level 5: mastery

To reach Level 5, *mastery*, they must not only demonstrate their autonomy in a variety of real, not training, contexts, but also be able to take a lead in new contexts and training programs themselves. They become the master practitioners, leading the company, or taking on the task of engaging and instructing others – running their own company or training program. A bonus talent will be a measure of enlightened opportunism, where they will identify potential needs and demands for applied theatre, or sites where the skills and structures of applied theatre could be valuable...and then work to make them happen! More than that they will be playing a mature part in developing the praxis of applied theatre and scholarship, and also creating networks of support. Following our ten-years-on interviews, we may say confidently that Baiyi and Tianxin have now reached the rarefied heights of Level 5: Mastery!

Conclusion: nurturing agency

Chapter 2 identified three generic aspects of learning – *personal, pedagogical,* and *reflective*. Although each aspect of generic learning is distinct and is mostly tacit in nature, the holistic capacities the learners have generated throughout directly contribute to their generic learning. This learning powerfully builds personal and professional agency. This supports their further learning within their practice at work, as well as sustaining further learning in applied theatre more generally. Key capacities to develop, along the way of participating in an applied theatre training program or when joining a human services company, are the capacity to feel, the capacity to express, the capacity to reflect and the capacity to practise. These grow respectively, from the experiential, presentational, propositional, and practical ways of knowing.

Each capacity to learn has a different level of impact on each of the three dimensions of generic learning – personal, pedagogical, and reflective. Obviously, even in a holistic learning program, some have more influence on individual learners than others.

Personal understanding capacity

Self-awareness, self-confidence, and social ability are three main types of personal learning that will develop. The capacity to feel is the critical foundational ability in personal learning. It enhances participants' level of awareness of their own inner feelings, self-limitations, and habitual behaviours as well as allowing them to notice and empathise with others' feelings. The capacity to express brings consciousness to trainees' thinking and feeling through active observation in action. That is followed by a capacity to articulate their knowledge and new capacities propositionally, in words and images. This automatically leads to the capacity to reflect, helping learners to ask why they acted in the way they did. Being mindfully aware of their own immediate feelings and emotions is an important source for reflection and to inform change for personal development.

The capacities that enhance trainees' self-awareness and social ability do not stop at the level of feeling and understanding but also help them to gain confidence to act according to their understanding and to try out something new, to explore the possibilities for change. They increase the degree of willingness and skills to practise, that build a culture of learning to make them feel safe and comfortable to express themselves. The training encourages expression via diverse aesthetic forms.

Pedagogical understanding capacity

Learners, whether trainees or new recruits, need to know about the people-centred, inclusive, participative, and dialogic pedagogy that is applied theatre. It takes 'being in' the pedagogy to fully understand it. Pedagogical learning that is generated through first-person experiential training is a kind of ritual knowledge that is gained, first and foremost, by and through the body. This starts with the learners' capacity to feel the personal benefits from 'living through' within the community of practice. Their expanding capacity to feel helps them to be actively aware of what they feel and others' feelings. They will observe how much they positively feel relaxed, equal, compassionate, respected, and empowered from their own experience. And they will also be able to feel the other group members' attitudinal and behavioural change through their empathic connection.

The central use of dialogical teaching builds learners' confidence in their ideas, and the skills to participate and to act expressively. It is also a means for them to acquire through embodied learning the pedagogical strategies. The capacity to reflect helps them consolidate their pedagogical experience and generalise the principles underpinning this teaching method.

Reflective understanding capacity

Reflectiveness is a capacity which can be learned or nurtured. Supported by all the other capacities, it is quite straightforward. It is – obviously – a direct outcome of reflective learning. Learning the personal and pedagogical skills all contributes to the development of a reflective capacity. Participants in applied theatre training go through the practice of applied theatre as an aesthetic, experience-based learning, grounded in feeling, expression, and practice.

Through this, participants learn how to reflect. This is an inner quality that is tacit in nature; but trainees and recruits will be able to consciously recognise this kind of generic learning when they can explain that they have gained a sense of being reflective. Then, reflection becomes a habitual skill that can be drawn upon or 'switched on' in life and at work. Their capacity to express has equipped them with diverse ways of reflection quite different from a 'normal' reliance on traditional conceptual thinking. Using imaginal patterns as a reflective source, particularly when confronting barriers and frustrations, allows the learners to reflect in action, and for their reflective learning to be seen in their practice.

Learning experience in applied theatre develops workers' and trainees' capacities to learn. The higher the level of their capacities, the more advanced the learner. The depth of their knowledge relies on the depth of their learning experience. We are not saying that all applied theatre experiences have the same quality to nurture learners' capacities; but the capacity to learn directly from them contributes to the generation of generic learning. They are crucial for nurturing the growth of the learner's personal and professional agency for sustainable learning, both in applied theatre and in professional fields beyond.

Note

1 Adapted, with acknowledgments, from O'Toole et al., 2015: 98–100.

References

Jarvis, P. (1994). Learning practical knowledge. *Journal of Further and Higher Education Research and Development*, *18*(1), 31–43.

Moon, J. A. (2004). *A handbook of reflective and experiential learning*. London: Routledge Falmer.

O'Toole, J., Au, Y.-M., Baldwin, A., Cahill, H., & Chinyowa, K. (2015). Capacity building theatre (and vice versa). In T. Prentki (Ed.). *Applied theatre: Development* (pp. 98–100). London: Bloomsbury.

Index

Entries in *italics* refer to titles and fictionalised names.

For Product Safety Concerns and Information please contact our EU
representative GPSR@taylorandfrancis.com Taylor & Francis Verlag GmbH,
Kaufingerstraße 24, 80331 München, Germany

Printed and bound by CPI Group (UK) Ltd, Croydon, CR0 4YY
08/06/2025
01897006-0018